Pilates for a
Flat Stomach

Other books by Anna Selby:

Pilates for Pregnancy
Banish Back Pain the Pilates Way

Anna Selby

Pilates for a
Flat Stomach

Core Strength in Just
15 Minutes a Day

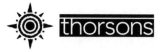

Thorsons
An Imprint of HarperCollins*Publishers*
77–85 Fulham Palace Road,
Hammersmith, London W6 8JB

The website is www.thorsonselement.com

-⚙- thorsons™

and *Thorsons* are trademarks of
HarperCollins*Publishers* Limited

First published 2003
10 9 8 7 6 5 4 3 2 1

A catalogue record for this book
is available from the British Library

ISBN 0 00 714127 0

Photography © Guy Hearn
Illustrations by PCA Creative

Printed and bound in Great Britain by
Martins The Printers Ltd, Berwick upon Tweed

Contents

How to Use This Book

There are many reasons why Pilates has become such a popular form of exercise. The main one, quite simply, is that it works. To get the most from the exercises in this book, however, you do need to do them properly. This means understanding the principles of the system and applying them so that you use your muscles in the most efficacious way.

I would always strongly recommend that you have at least a few lessons with an experienced Pilates teacher, rather than launch into uncharted waters on your own! We all develop little quirks of posture and movement that over time can turn into bad habits – so sometimes you may think you are doing an exercise correctly when in fact you are using all the wrong muscles in an effort to simulate the photograph in the book. Because Pilates is such a precise science, you need to become very aware of how your body works and how to use it in the best possible way. A good teacher will help you do this. My first Pilates teacher was Dreas Reyneke and, after around three sessions at his London studio, I found I was walking down the street in a completely different way – feeling lighter, looser, more poised and more relaxed. I hadn't even been aware that tension had been bunching up my muscles and joints in various parts of my anatomy!

As with any exercise regime, if you have any concerns whatsoever about your health, you should consult your doctor before you begin. With this particular book, this applies tenfold if you have any back problems. The strength of the back and the abdomen are closely interrelated and I would strongly recommend anyone with back problems to work thoroughly through the first level of exercises before going on to the second – and to leave out the third level altogether. And, if ever you feel any strain or pain in the back, or if the muscles start to bulge or quiver during an exercise, always stop immediately. Your muscles are not yet strong enough for what you are trying to do; strengthen them with exercises you can do without straining and come back to the harder ones when you're ready.

The book is divided into three main sections, the exercises becoming progressively harder. You don't need to be on to the most strenuous exercises, though, to achieve your goal. Because you use your muscles in a very precise and controlled manner in Pilates, you will start to

Pilates for a Flat Stomach

strengthen and flatten your stomach muscles from the very beginning. In fact, you can stay permanently at stage one and get a result, providing you do the exercises thoroughly and regularly. The later exercises will give you added strength but if they are too much of a strain for your abdominal muscles, that strain will be transferred to your back – with the inevitable consequences of back pain or strain. So, the underlying principle with this book is to take it gently and work through each stage until you can perform each exercise fluently and accurately, and only then to go on to the next stage.

What is Pilates?

The Pilates method originated around one hundred years ago near Düsseldorf in Germany when a frail child called Joseph Pilates took up body-building to increase his strength. At the time he was thought to be prone to tuberculosis, as well as being generally weak and sickly but, so successful was the programme he devised, that by the age of 14, he was posing as a model for anatomical drawings.

He went on to become a keen sportsman – gymnast, skier, boxer, diver – and even a circus performer. In 1912, he left his native Germany and moved to England where, at the outbreak of the First World War, he was interned as a enemy alien. Pilates used his enforced leisure to develop his method of attaining peak physical fitness.

Pilates called his new system 'muscle contrology' and, in it, he aimed to bring about the complete co-ordination of body, mind and spirit by working with – not on or against – the body's muscles. After the war, he returned briefly to Germany and then moved to New York, where his method was an immediate success, particularly with dancers such as Martha Graham and George Balanchine, the founder of the New York City Ballet. It remained something of a secret amongst dancers until comparatively recently when sportsmen, actors and the public began to discover it. The popularity of Pilates has soared over the last few years.

THE ORIGINAL PILATES METHOD

Much of Pilates' early work was based on the rehabilitation of ill or injured people. During his internment, when Pilates worked as a nurse, he had experimented devising an exercise regime using springs attached to hospital beds, so that patients could begin to work on toning their muscles even before they could get up. Springs used as resistance were the cornerstone of the method and Pilates designed a machine that he called the 'universal reformer', a sliding horizontal bed that could be used with up to four springs, according to the exercise and the strength of the individual. On this machine, one could perform pliés and other exercises but without putting any weight on the joints (and so beneficial for those with injuries or other joint problems) and against resistance (so that the muscles would be worked harder).

Pilates developed several other machines for his New York studio and these have been adapted and used around the world ever since. More recently, the principles of the Pilates method have been adapted for use without machines and this system has become particularly popular. It is this version of Pilates that has been used in this book.

The Pilates Principles

The Pilates method has changed substantially over the decades but its underlying principles remain the same. One of these is that Pilates is, quite simply, the thinking person's exercise. Unlike the kind of workout that involves jumping around to loud music, where your main priority is to keep up, in Pilates every movement is carefully controlled for maximum effect. To work, it requires concentration. For each and every exercise there are questions you need to ask yourself. Is the navel drawn towards the spine? Is the heel in the correct position? Is the neck long and aligned with the spine? Are you doing the correct breathing?

In the Pilates method, the placing and movement of every part of your body counts and the body works as an integrated system. The more you use your body correctly during exercise, the more you will use it correctly in everything you do. Your posture improves and the headaches, tight, contracted muscles and tensions that arise from poor posture all fade away.

Interestingly, all this concentration does not leave you mentally drained or exhausted. On the contrary, it is a profoundly relaxing method of exercise, and its slow, rhythmic movements are a stress relief in themselves and leave most people feeling simultaneously calm and energized.

In the long term, the effect of Pilates on the body is to give your muscles a long, toned shape rather than bulk. Think of a dancer's body, rather than a gym fanatic's.

THE PRINCIPLES

Before you begin the exercises, it is important to understand the theory that underlies the Pilates method. These are the essential principles to bear in mind whenever you exercise:

- **Concentration**: As I have already said, concentration is fundamental to this way of exercising. This is not only because it is important that every part of your body is moving or positioned correctly – a part of a synchronized whole. It is also because, when you concentrate on your body in this way, it actually leads your mind away from any immediate concerns or anxieties and is profoundly relaxing.

- **The breath**: The way you breathe is vitally important within the Pilates method – you should breathe deeply, rhythmically and to your full capacity. The other point to remember is *when* you breathe. In Pilates exercises, you breathe out with the effort. This is not the way most people breathe – in fact, it's the opposite – but it does help you to relax into a movement. If you breathe in for the effort of an exercise, you will automatically tense up.

- **The girdle of strength**: According to Joseph Pilates, the 'girdle of strength' was essential for all exercise. This 'girdle' incorporates three main areas – the back, the abdomen and the buttocks. The upper back can be a major seat of tension, but when you learn to move the arms correctly (from the middle of the back rather than the shoulders), this tension will disappear. Nearly every exercise in this book begins by drawing the navel gently towards the spine. This strengthens the abdominal muscles to ensure you will have the flat stomach you want, and it protects the back against undue strain during the exercise. The third element in this girdle of strength is the buttock muscles. By engaging and squeezing these during the exercises, you not only tone the muscles themselves but you also bring the body into perfect alignment, improving the posture and protecting the back from strain or injury.

- **Flowing movements**: Unlike many forms of exercise, Pilates admits no sudden, jerky movements. Instead, one position flows as slowly and naturally as possible into the next. You move rhythmically, your pace set by your own breathing, and this warms the muscles and makes them lengthen out rather than bunch and bulk up. Moving slowly also gives you time to become aware of each part of your body so that you perform all the exercises with precision and in a co-ordinated way.

- **Relaxation**: This is an important element of the Pilates method, particularly as the stresses and strains of modern living can result in bunched-up, tense muscles that in turn lead to headaches, strains and injuries. The relaxation exercises at the end of each session are very important. Make sure you do them to restore flagging energy levels and, just as crucially, to induce a tranquil state of mind.

Pilates for a Flat Stomach

How Pilates Helps You Get a Flat Stomach

A flat stomach is not so much an aim of Pilates' technique as its inevitable side-effect. As has already been explained in the Pilates Principles, the girdle of strength is the key to the technique and, of all the muscles in the body, the abdominals play the greatest part in creating it. The girdle of strength gives you your core strength and it is from this centre that all your movements should originate.

There are four layers of abdominal muscles, criss-crossing the body over the front, sides and back. They are the means by which you can bend and twist but, even more importantly, when developed and used correctly, they protect the spine and the internal muscles from strain and injury. When they are strong, they give all of your movements support and flexibility. Unfortunately, though, the sedentary lifestyle most of us have nowadays means not only are these muscles not strong, we are often barely aware of them.

The four layers of abdominal muscles form a girdle (hence Pilates' name for them) between the rib cage and the pelvis. The top layer (*see opposite*) is the rectus abdominis, running vertically down the front of the body from the sternum to the pelvis. It draws the front of the pelvis upwards and is important for maintaining posture. Divided into four

Pilates for a Flat Stomach

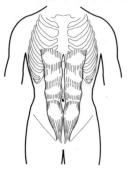

The rectus abdominis muscles

sections, it is also the muscle people tend to notice the most – and is responsible for visible six-packs!

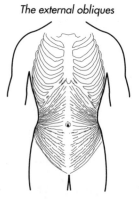

The external obliques

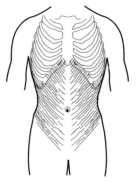

The internal obliques

The external obliques run diagonally from just below the sternum and wrap around the waist. The internal obliques are underneath them, and run diagonally from the lower ribs down to the pelvis. Both sets of oblique muscles are used in turning and bending the body.

The transversus abdominis muscle

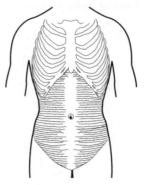

The deepest layer is the transversus abdominis. This runs horizontally around the waist to the back and down in front of the hips towards the pelvis. This is an often forgotten muscle and strengthening it will not only create a strong, flat stomach, it will also give support and stability to the lower back.

As you do the exercises in this book, you will become aware of these layers of muscle and start to strengthen them. However, it is not only when you exercise that you should be using them. One of the most important benefits of Pilates' technique is that it re-educates your body, how you hold it and move it in everyday life. So, the instruction to 'draw the navel to the spine' that starts off almost every exercise that follows is just as relevant to your normal standing posture or the way you walk.

Posture is covered in more detail on pages 135–38 and in the exercises in the following section, Applying the Principles. But, even before you begin to exercise, it is worth taking a few moments to see how just this simple movement can change the way you feel and look.

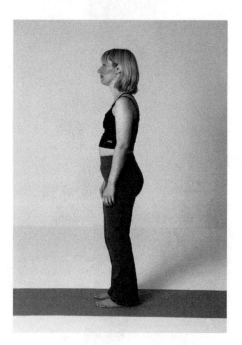

Stand in front of a mirror in your normal posture. Now make a few minor adjustments. Check that your feet are flat on the floor, hip-width apart, with the toes pointing forwards.

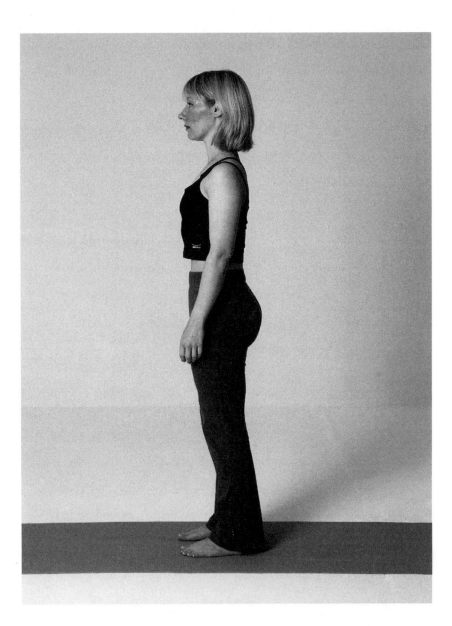

Pilates for a Flat Stomach

Now, without changing anything else, engage your abdominal muscles so that your navel simultaneously lifts slightly upwards and draws back towards the spine. You should feel that the lower back loses just a little of its natural curve and feels more supported. Your stomach will automatically look flatter and, lifting up out of the waist, the waist too becomes more defined. You will also probably look as if you have lengthened out slightly – you might even grow an inch! If you now also let your shoulders drop down and feel your neck relaxed and the top of your chest soft and open, you are getting pretty close to your ideal posture. The effect is not just cosmetic, either. This kind of posture gives you strength and stability, as well as protecting your back.

This simple exercise should give you an idea of how much you can achieve by posture alone. The next section, Applying the Principles, shows you in more detail how to achieve correct alignment and, just as important, how you use breathing in Pilates. Basically, in Pilates, you exhale on the effort – the opposite of many forms of sports and exercise when you breathe in on the movement. The inhalation in Pilates is used as a form of preparation and you do the work on the exhalation. This encourages your muscles to lengthen during the exercise and creates muscles that are strong but not bunched – instead, they become long and lean, like a dancer's.

Applying the Principles

The exercises in this section are designed to help you find your correct posture and alignment so that you will be using the right muscles in the exercises that follow and so get the maximum benefit from them. It is worth coming back to these exercises on a regular basis just to check your alignment, and as a warm-up for the exercises in the later sections.

Roll Down Against the Wall

This exercise mobilizes and places the spine in its correct alignment. The more slowly you do this exercise, the better. Try to feel each vertebra as you draw it away or place it against the wall. You will find it is your abdominal muscles that do the work of controlling your body's alignment – but you should also check that there is no tension anywhere (particularly in your neck, shoulders or back).

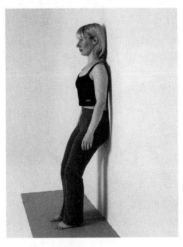

Stand 12–18 inches away from the wall with the knees slightly bent and the feet hip-width apart, toes facing forwards. Measure out the entire length of your spine against the wall (leaving no gaps), with the head held high on a long neck and the shoulders relaxed. Your arms hang comfortably at your sides. Draw your navel gently to the spine.

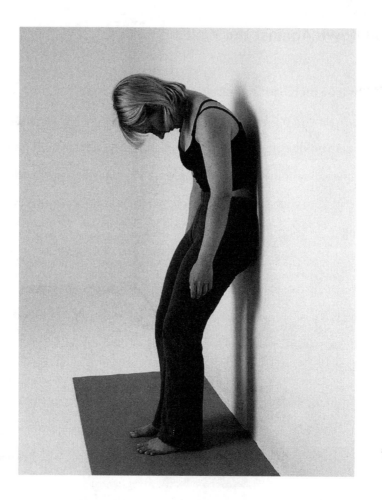

Breathe in and, as you breathe out, pull your navel towards your spine and drop your chin to your chest, feeling the stretch all the way through the neck and upper back. As you begin to mobilize the spine, the arms will move naturally – just let them hang, don't try to place them.

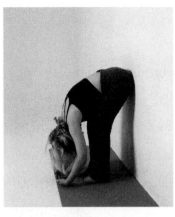

Let the curve deepen so the back peels away from the wall in a long, relaxed curve, head and arms hanging until only the buttocks are touching the wall. Breathe naturally for a few moments as your body hangs upside down and releases into the stretch.

On the next out-breath, check that your navel is still drawn towards the spine and the pelvic floor muscles are pulled up, and rotate from the pelvis to bring yourself back to a standing position, feeling your back touch the wall vertebra by vertebra. As the back unrolls, feel the shoulders drop down naturally. The head comes in line with the spine, last of all. Check that your back is long, your neck and shoulders are relaxed and your 'girdle of strength' is working. Repeat the whole thing three times.

Finding Neutral

The previous exercise begins to mobilize the spine and work the abdominal muscles. This exercise builds on that by developing awareness of where your spine and abdominal muscles should be placed when you are exercising. This placement is vital to the accurate performance of the exercises that follow in the later stages.

Lie on your back with your knees bent and your feet flat on the floor, parallel (toes facing straight ahead) and in line with your hips. You can put a thin cushion under your head if it makes you more comfortable. Your arms should be relaxed by your sides with no tension in the shoulders or, if you prefer to feel the extent of the movement more strongly, place your hands on your abdomen.

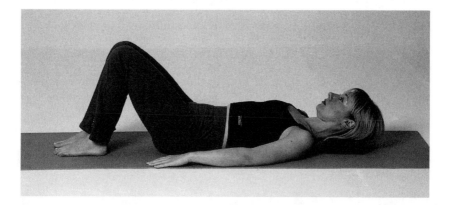

You will find there is a natural curve in your back and – the extent varies from individual to individual – some of your spine will not be in contact with the floor. Now, curl your buttocks up and feel your spine flatten out along the floor. This is a pelvic tilt and, while it is needed in some exercises, in others it would distort the correct working of the muscles.

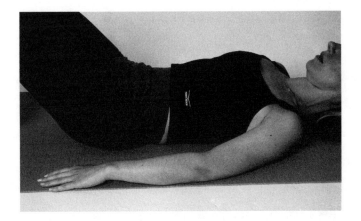

Now, replace your buttocks on the floor, curving in the opposite direction so that your back hollows out and widens the gap between your spine and the floor. Your abdomen will bulge out. This is a position you should never use – though it is a common postural problem – in which you cannot work your abdominal muscles and you can put a potentially dangerous strain on your back.

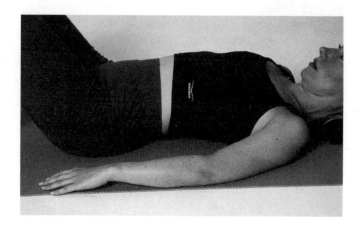

Return to the first position and feel your spine long and relaxed with a slight arch around the small of the back. Draw your abdominal muscles gently towards the spine, but without distorting it or moving the pelvis, so they are held lightly but firmly. This is your neutral position and, unless the exercise you are doing entails a pelvic tilt, this is the placement in which you will perform most of the movements.

Breathing Exercise

In Pilates exercises, you use the breath in a very specific way. For the most part, all movement and effort takes place on the out-breath, while on the in-breath you are either stretching, preparing or relaxing. Breathing in on the effort results in tension and bunching in the muscles, whereas when you make the effort on the out-breath, in the Pilates way, you elongate the muscles. This is particularly relevant to the strengthening and defining of the abdominal muscles – however, you must breathe slowly and deeply for the best effects. Many of us breathe shallowly and rapidly, our lungs failing to reach their potential to fill completely. This exercise helps you to breathe deeply, allowing the oxygen to circulate more efficiently through your body, and developing your awareness of the link between the abdominal muscles and the breath.

P.T.O. ➤

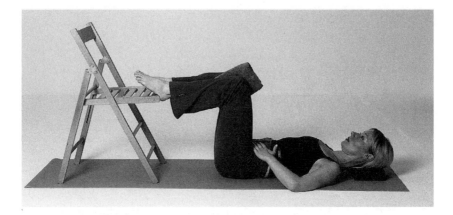

Lie on your back with a small cushion underneath your head and your feet up on a chair so that your knees form a right angle. Put a small cushion or rolled-up towel between your knees and keep it in place throughout. Check that your back is long and straight and there is no tension in the neck or shoulders. Place your hands on your abdomen so that your middle fingers are barely touching. As you breathe in, the inhalation should reach all the way down to the abdomen and part the fingers. As you breathe out, the fingers meet again. Try not to exaggerate this movement and do not push the abdomen out or arch in the back, but keep the spine neutral. Just try to feel the breath filling your body and relax. Repeat for 10 breaths. Use this type of breathing whenever you do a relaxation exercise.

Now place the hands on the ribs. Breathe in and, as you breathe out, engage the abdominal muscles and draw the navel towards the spine and feel the lower back lengthen out against the floor. Keep the abdominal muscles engaged as you take 10 long, slow breaths, feeling the breath fill and extend the ribs so that they expand outwards a little. With the abdominal muscles engaged, you will not be able to take the breath into the abdomen and this is the way that you should breathe in all of the exercises – virtually every one – in which the navel is drawn to the spine. You can also do this exercise sitting on a chair in front of a mirror so that you can observe the change in the body when you breathe into the ribs.

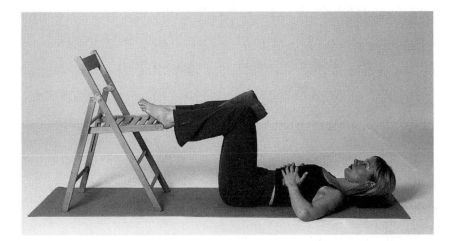

Stage One Exercises

This first level of exercises helps you to locate and mobilize all of the muscle groups you need to achieve your goal of a flat stomach. It is very important to take as long as you need getting the exercises in this section right before you go on to the next one. Pilates is a very precise form of exercise, so make sure you are using the correct muscles and, whenever possible, practise in front of a mirror so you can check your posture. In particular, make sure the right part of the body is doing the work – almost always the abdominal muscles, sometimes in conjunction with others, such as the thigh or buttock muscles. However, it is never the back, shoulders or neck that should be feeling the strain – if they do, stop immediately and try to work out what you are doing wrong. It may simply be that your abdominal muscles are not yet strong enough for a particular exercise. So, do those that you can and build up your muscles' strength gradually. If you can, it is a good idea to go to some classes with a qualified Pilates teacher, who will be able to spot mistakes that you may notice.

The Scoop

The Scoop is a pelvic tilt that builds your awareness of and works the abdominal muscles. Make sure you begin the exercise with a neutral spine and work slowly through the base of the spine, feeling the interrelation between the abdominals and the back.

Lie on your back on the floor with your knees raised to the ceiling and your feet flat on the floor, hip-width apart. Check that your back is long and there is no tension in the shoulders, neck or face. Place your arms a little apart from your sides.

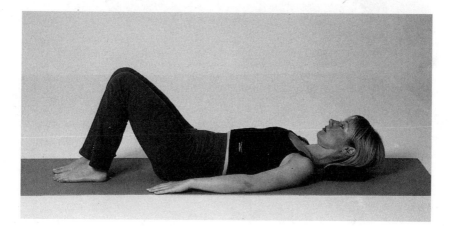

Breathe in and, as you breathe out, draw the navel to the spine, squeeze the pelvic floor and the low buttock muscles and feel the abdomen hollow out into a shallow scoop. This movement takes place only in the lower body – your upper body should remain still and without any tension.

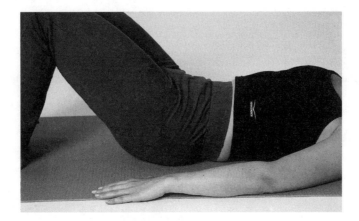

Repeat up to 10 times, each time trying to extend the movement. If your abdominal muscles are strong enough, you can curl up the lower buttocks very slightly from the floor. Keep the lower back on the floor at all times, though, and if you feel any strain, don't try to take the buttocks off the floor either.

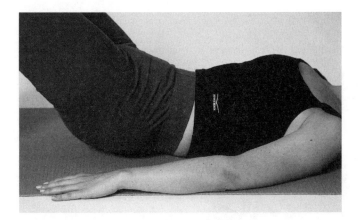

Hip Rolls

This exercise is designed to release tension from the back and neck and it should feel particularly good after the last exercise. Your abdominal muscles are 'carrying' the weight of your legs, so don't take them so far that it puts a strain on the back or abdominals themselves.

Lie on your back with your feet hip-width apart and your knees raised. Check that your neck and spine are long and relaxed.

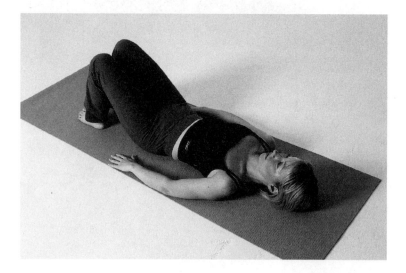

Breathe in and, as you breathe out, draw your navel towards your spine without distorting the back, and roll your knees gently to one side. Take them only as far as they will go without your buttocks coming off the floor.

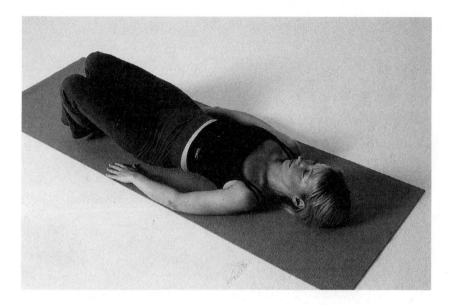

Breathe in to return to the centre and, as you breathe out, roll your knees to the other side. Repeat up to 10 times on each side.

Curl-ups

This exercise is the opposite of the Scoop – it mobilizes the top of the spine. However, it uses the abdominal muscles to do the work in just the same way, strengthening and placing them against the spine.

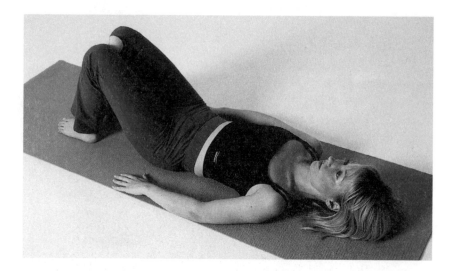

Lie on your back with your knees raised, the feet slightly apart and flat on the floor. Place a rolled-up towel or a tennis ball between your knees and keep it in place by squeezing the thighs together throughout the exercise. Feel the spine long and relaxed. Tuck your chin in a little to release and lengthen the back of the neck. Check that your shoulders and neck are relaxed, too. Place your hands on the front of your thighs.

Pilates for a Flat Stomach

Take a long, slow breath in and, as you breathe out, draw the navel gently towards the spine and squeeze the lower buttock and the pelvic floor muscles. Walk your fingers up the front of your thighs so that your head, neck and upper back start to curl up from the floor, very slowly, vertebra by vertebra. Don't lift any further than your shoulder blades – they should stay in contact with the floor. At the furthest point, check that your shoulders and neck are still relaxed and your abdominal muscles have not popped out or started to tremble.

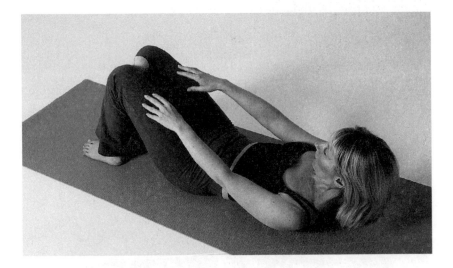

When you have lifted yourself up as far as is comfortable, take another in-breath and, as you breathe out, lower the back down in exactly the same way, trying to feel each vertebra as you place it on the floor. Repeat 5–10 times, depending on the strength of your abdominals.

Oblique Curl-ups

This exercise is very similar to the previous one except that it uses the abdominal muscles at the side rather than the centre of your body. You may find this exercise harder than the last one as these muscles are often used less than the central ones. If your abdominal muscles pop out or start to tremble or if you feel back pain at any time, stop immediately.

Lie on your back as in the previous exercise, with a rolled-up towel or a tennis ball between your knees. As before, keep it in place by squeezing the inner thighs together throughout the exercise. Make sure the shoulders and neck stay relaxed throughout – check each time you start to curl up.

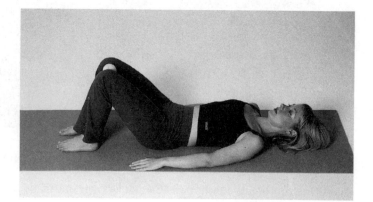

Breathe in and, as you breathe out, draw the navel gently to the spine and start to curl up the head and neck, turning the body so that the right shoulder points towards the left knee. Don't lead with the elbow – keep the elbows wide. Move slowly and go only as far as you can without the abdominal muscles bulging or trembling.

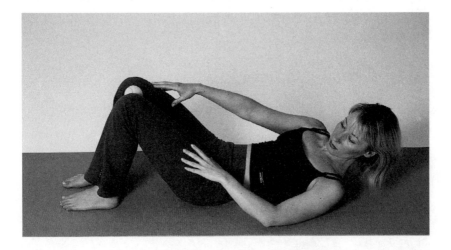

Breathe in and, on the out-breath, curl back down to the floor. Relax for a moment, check there is no tension (particularly in the neck or shoulders), then repeat on the other side, curling the right shoulder towards the left knee. Repeat, alternating from side to side, up to five times.

Side Rolls

This exercise is similar to the Hip Rolls on page 24. Now, though, you do it with a tennis ball to help you keep the knees together and level. You will not be able to take the knees as far as in the Hip Rolls. The important element here is to control the movement and do it as slowly as possible.

Lie on your back with your knees raised and feel your spine long and straight on the floor. Place your arms on the floor at a 45-degree angle to your body, palms facing upwards, with no tension in the shoulders or neck. Place a tennis ball between your knees with your feet the same distance apart.

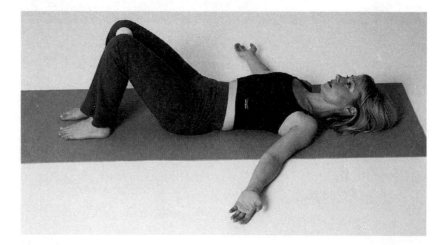

Breathe in and, as you breathe out, start to roll your knees slowly in one direction, your head in the other. Your feet will turn on to their sides but they should not come off the floor completely. Keep both shoulders on the floor throughout. Use your abdominal muscles to control the movement, and don't let your back arch.

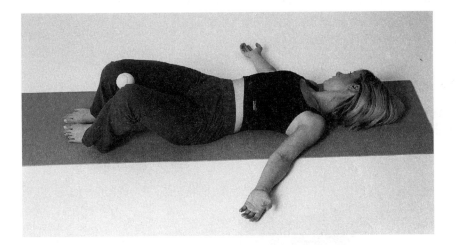

When you have turned as far as you can without straining, breathe in. As you breathe out, come back to the centre, again using the abdominal muscles to roll the ribs, then the back, and then the buttocks on to the floor. Check that your shoulders have not lifted or tensed and correct them if they have. Now repeat in the other direction slowly. Repeat up to 10 times.

Leg Stretches

This is one of the most famous of Pilates exercises. The original is tough (see Single Leg Stretch, Stage Two, on pages 56–7) and it has been adapted here to introduce you to the movement without straining. Don't go on to the Stage Two version until you can do this one with ease.

Lie on your back with your feet flat on the floor and your knees raised. Now draw your knees to your chest, keeping them apart to make a V-shape towards your toes. Check that your back is flat on the floor and your neck and shoulders are relaxed.

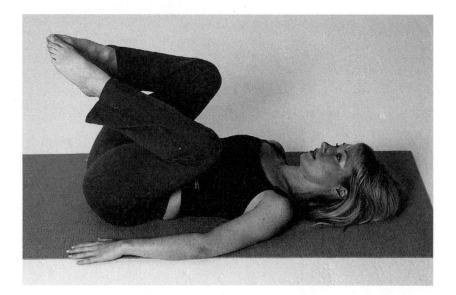

Breathe in and bring one knee up towards your chest. Then, as you breathe out, draw the navel to the spine, making sure the whole spine is on the floor, and stretch the second leg vertically up into the air with a pointed toe. Check that the spine is still elongated along the floor and there is no tension in the neck or shoulders.

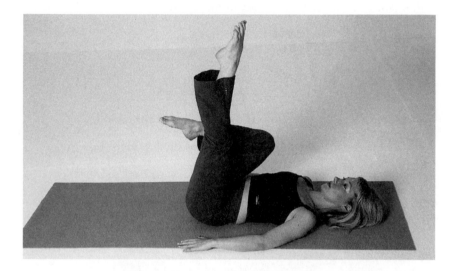

Take another long full breath and, as you breathe out, change the legs so that the second leg is drawn in towards your chest and the first is stretched out. Always keep the whole back on the floor. If you start to hollow out the small of the back, your leg is too low – make sure it is 90 degrees to the floor. If you feel any discomfort stop immediately. Alternate 5–10 times on each side.

The Cat

If you felt any tension during the last exercise, this one will help to release it. It stretches and releases the back and the best way of doing it is as slowly and smoothly as possible, allowing one position to blend into the next. If you have any back problems, however, only do the first two positions.

If possible, position yourself next to a mirror so you can check that your back is completely flat. Position yourself on your hands and knees, with your knees hip-width apart, and check that your shoulders, hips and knees are in a straight alignment. Try to make your back perfectly flat with no tension in the neck and your head relaxed in line with the spine.

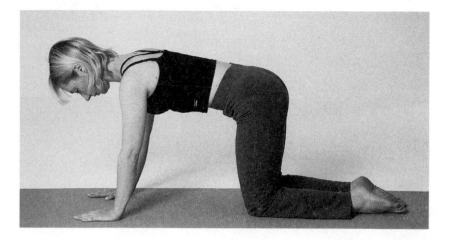

Breathe in and, as you breathe out, gently draw the navel back towards the spine so that your back arches upwards and your head drops down between the arms. Breathe in and return to position one.

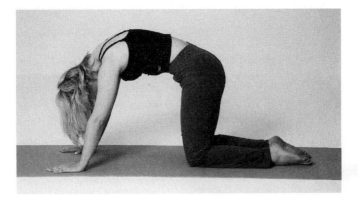

Breathe out and arch your back the other way so that it hollows out with your head and your bottom the highest points of your body. Breathe in and return to position one. Repeat 5–10 times.

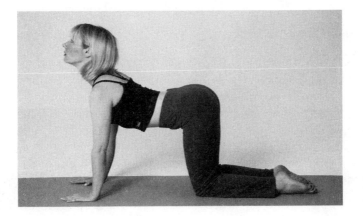

Simple Double Leg Stretch

This Double Leg Stretch has been adapted from the original version (see page 92) as an easier introduction to one of the tougher Pilates' sequential movements. It's not too easy, though, as your abdominal muscles have to be strong enough to carry the weight of both your legs. Make sure you stretch your legs upwards at 90 degrees to the floor – the lower your legs, the harder the exercise is to do. Keep checking that your abdominals aren't bulging out or trembling with the effort. If they do either, stop immediately.

Lie on your back with your knees bent, feet flat on the floor and your back long and straight. Place your hands, with your fingers lightly clasped, behind your head. Don't use your hands to pull your head up, though, and keep checking throughout that the shoulders and neck are free from tension.

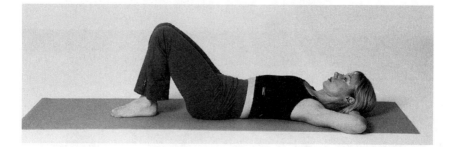

Breathe in and, as you breathe out, draw the navel to the spine and bend the knees to a right angle, the feet softly pointed.

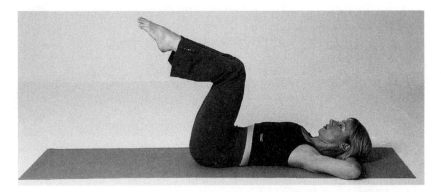

Breathe out, curl the head and neck up from the floor and straighten the legs up towards the ceiling. If it is uncomfortable you can leave the knees slightly bent.

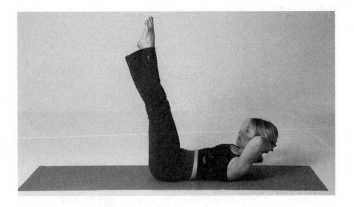

Breathe in and, as you breathe out, bend the knees back to right angles and lower the head to the floor. Repeat up to 10 times.

Child's Pose

This is actually a yoga pose rather than a Pilates exercise but it is perfect for releasing and stretching the back after the previous exercise.

Kneel down on the floor and sit back as much as possible on your heels. Bend forwards, place your forehead on the floor or a small cushion and stretch your arms out as flat on the floor as you can. Check there is no tension anywhere in the body (the neck, shoulders and back are all potential danger spots) and feel a stretch for the whole length of your spine.

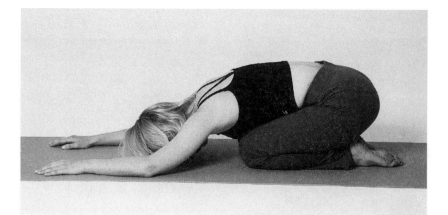

Take one arm back and lay it down at your side, palm uppermost. If it is more comfortable, turn your head so that your cheek rather than your forehead is against the floor.

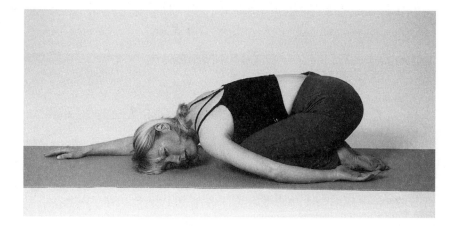

Now take the other arm and lay it down next to you in the same way. Relax into the pose for two minutes, or longer if you have the time.

Pillow Squeeze

This is another famous Pilates exercise that has a number of benefits and is particularly good for relaxing the lower back at the end of your exercise session. You will need a pillow or cushion for this exercise – the firmer it is, the harder you will have to work.

Lie on your back with your knees raised up and your feet flat on the floor. Place your arms by your sides, palms down. Check your shoulders and neck are relaxed and, if you are at all uncomfortable or the neck feels arched away from the floor, place a small pillow underneath your head. Breathe in, pulling up the pelvic floor muscles.

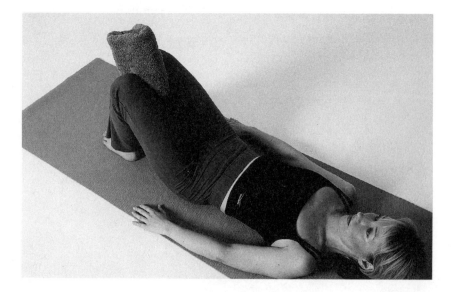

As you breathe out, draw the navel to the spine and squeeze the cushion with your knees, taking care not to let your back arch or tension to creep into the back, neck or shoulders. The abdominal muscles should be engaged but the only part of the body that should be moving is the knees.

Breathe in to release and repeat up to 10 times.

Relaxation Sequence

After the exercises, it is important for you to relax; and even a short relaxation will make a big difference to your stress levels and overall health. The relaxation takes place in what is known in yoga as the corpse pose. Many people find it helpful to record the following instructions on tape and play it while they do the relaxation. If you do this, ensure you speak very slowly, repeating each instruction several times. During the relaxation, your body temperature will drop, so now is the time to cover yourself with a blanket or to put on an extra layer of clothing, especially socks as your feet can get cold. I recommend finishing each of the stages in the book with this relaxation session.

Lie down on the floor with your spine long and your arms close to your sides, palms uppermost. It may seem more natural to face the palms down, but when they are facing up, the upper back and shoulders are lowered and not tensed and your back is more comfortable on the floor. Close your eyes and give yourself a few moments in which to become aware of the weight of your whole body, softening and spreading out on the floor after the exertions of exercising and stretching. Roll the head from side to side to check there is no tension in the neck.

Pilates for a Flat Stomach

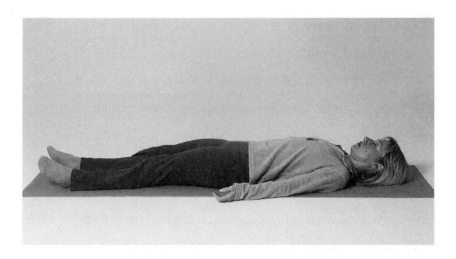

Starting at your toes, begin to feel the relaxation spreading through your body, moving upwards like a wave. Spend time on each tiny part, putting all your concentration into each area of your body in turn, first the toes, then the feet and ankles.

Feel the wave spreading up into your legs, through the shins and calves, the knees and into the thighs. Let your legs roll outwards from the hips, completely relaxed. Let the hips and buttocks go – there is often a surprising amount of tension stored here. The whole body softens and the effect now reaches the abdomen, which drops down further against the back, while the lower spine relaxes further into the floor.

The stomach, the waist and the ribs all expand and soften. Your breathing is now probably quite light. As the softening, relaxing wave flows through the torso and into the back, they fall deeper into the floor. The relaxation comes up into the shoulders and neck and out along the arms to the very ends of the fingers. The back of the neck is almost touching the floor, the scalp softens, almost loose against the skull, and the whole face – the jaw, the chin, the throat, the cheeks – melt away. The lips part and the tongue rests gently behind the lower teeth. The eyes sink softly back into the head and the temples and forehead smooth out.

Your whole body is at rest. Enjoy this sensation; be aware of it. As thoughts come into your mind, watch them and see them float away like clouds in a summer sky. Any doubts or worries can float away in the same way as the physical tension has left your body. Stay in this place for a few minutes. Now see the sun in your sky and feel its life-giving light and warmth. Feel the air around you and, as you take a deep breath in, feel that you are drinking in from the sun's vast source of energy, making you calmer and stronger.

Now begin to deepen the breath, letting the ribs expand and the lungs fill. After three breaths, begin to feel your toes and fingers coming to life. Wriggle them. Still with your eyes closed, lift your arms above your head and stretch your arms and legs away from each other. When you are ready, roll onto your side and open your eyes. Give yourself a few moments before you get up.

Stage Two Exercises

Start the second level of exercises only when you can do the first stage correctly and without any straining. Incorporate all of the principles from Stage One to the way you work in this more difficult stage and, if any exercise is too much of a strain, particularly if it affects the back, go back to the easier version in Stage One.

This section extends the exercises from the previous one, using other parts of the body as weights to work the abdominal muscles. It also introduces a new, deep abdominal movement from contemporary dance – the contraction.

Pelvic Tilts

This exercise builds on the Scoop from the previous stage but it is harder as you now have your feet raised up on a chair. It is a good idea to use the Scoop (see page 21) as a warm-up for this one and build up the repetitions gradually. As with the earlier version, it is important that you don't try to come up too far. If your lower back begins to arch or you feel any back pain, or if the abdominal or thigh muscles quiver, come back down to the floor. Keep the movement slow and controlled throughout.

Lie on your back on the floor with your feet on a stable chair. Check that your back is long and there is no tension in the shoulders, neck or face. Place your arms a little apart from your sides, palms down.

Breathe in and, as you breathe out, draw the navel to the spine, squeeze the pelvic floor and the lower buttock muscles and feel the abdomen hollow out into a shallow scoop. This movement takes place only in the lower body – your upper body should remain still and without any tension.

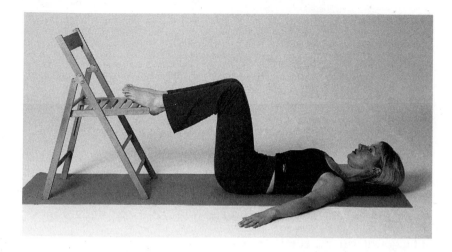

Keeping the scooped-out shape, curl up the lower buttocks from the floor. Lower and repeat up to 10 times.

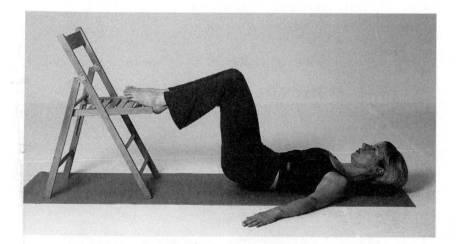

Curl-ups

As with the previous exercise, these curl-ups build on those you did in Stage One. Take them slowly at first, though, or you may find the effort is in your back rather than your abs – and that will not only defeat the object, it will give you back problems as well. Always prepare as you did for the pelvic tilt, engaging the abdominal and lower buttock muscles. And, if you feel any strain in the back or your abdominal muscles quiver or bulge out with the effort, it means you have come up too far, so take it lower until you feel stronger.

Lie on your back with your knees raised and your feet flat on the floor. Place a cushion or a rolled-up towel between your knees to remind you to keep your legs still and check there is no tension in your neck or shoulders. Place your hands behind your neck lightly – don't use them to hoist yourself up during the exercise.

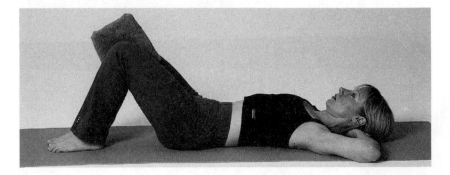

Breathe in and, as you breathe out, draw the navel to the spine and engage the low buttock muscles. Start to curl your head and shoulders off the floor. If you can only raise your head to start with, don't worry – just keep working at this level until you are stronger. The most important thing to check is that your abs are not bulging or quivering with the effort. If they are try the exercise lower. Another sign you have come too far off the floor is if the neck and shoulders start to tense up. The neck should be long, the shoulders down and you should be looking straight ahead, rather than down to your body.

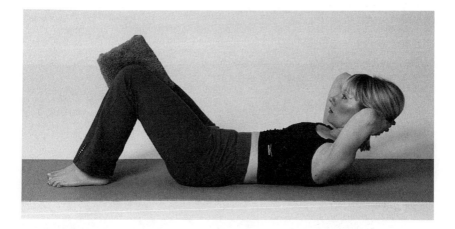

When you have come up as far as you can without straining, breathe in and roll down to the floor. Check for tension, especially in the upper body or the jaw. Rest if necessary and then repeat up to 10 times.

Oblique Curl-ups

As in the previous exercise, curl up only as far as you can without feeling the strain in your back or neck.

Lie on your back with your knees raised and your feet flat on the floor, as in the previous exercise, but this time with only your right hand behind your head and the left arm down by your side. Check that your shoulders and neck are relaxed.

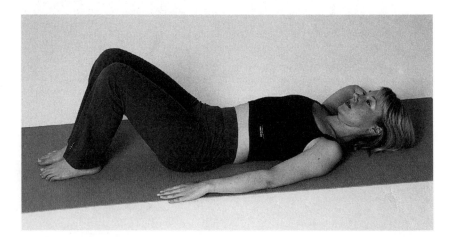

Breathe in and, as you breathe out, draw the navel to the spine, engage the low buttock muscles and curl up, taking your right shoulder towards your left knee. As in the previous exercise, if the abdominal muscles start to bulge or quiver, if there is any strain in the back or tension in the neck or shoulders, you are coming up too far from the floor.

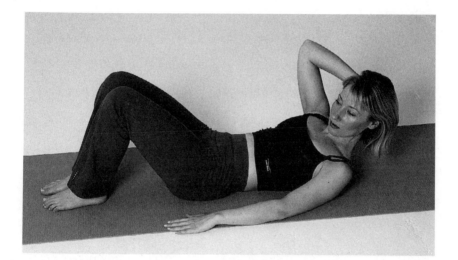

Breathe in and lower to the floor. Repeat on each side, up to 10 times.

After the last three exercises, all of which are hard work for the abdominal muscles, relax into the Child's Pose (see page 38) before you continue the session.

Leg Lifts

This exercise uses your leg as a weight but the work is done by your abdominal muscles. It is best to practise this one with your back against a wall to ensure you don't arch it.

Lie on your right side, preferably against a wall with a big cushion beneath your left leg, and smaller ones to support your waist and between your head and arm. Make sure that your back is flat against the wall and stretch out your right arm parallel to your spine, placing a cushion between it and your head. Bend your right leg and flex the foot of your left leg on the cushions.

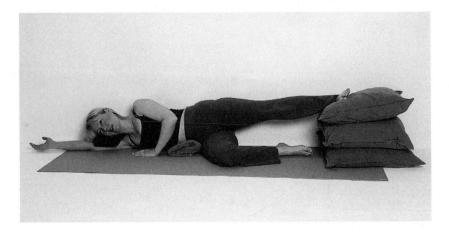

Place your left hand on your left hip and take a long breath in. As you breathe out, draw the navel gently to the spine and feel the shoulder blades draw down and the neck lengthen. Lengthen out along your left side and bring up your left leg in a low lift, making sure the whole leg – foot, knee and hip – is facing forwards. The feeling to aim for is a long stretch rather than an actual lift.

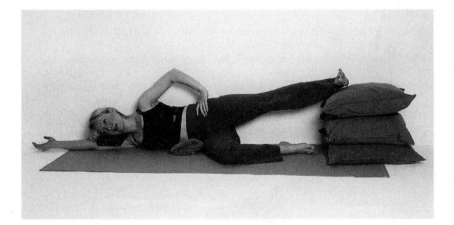

Do 5–10 lifts and then repeat on the other side.

Single Leg Stretches

This exercise extends the leg stretching from Stage One (see page 32). Because your leg is lower, this exercise is more demanding – but only take the leg as low as you can without the abdominal muscles popping out or the strain transferring to your back.

Lie on your back with your feet flat on the floor and your knees raised. Now draw your knees to your chest, keeping them apart to make a V-shape towards your toes. Check that your back is flat on the floor and your neck and shoulders are relaxed.

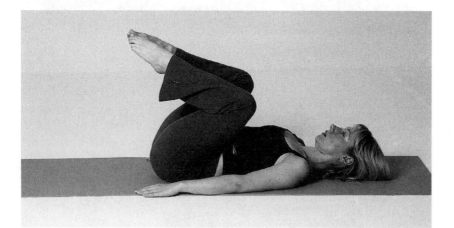

Breathe in and, as you breathe out, draw the navel to the spine, making sure the whole spine is on the floor. Bring the left knee closer to your chest and stretch out the right leg in front of you with a pointed toe. Check that the spine is still elongated along the floor and there is no tension in the neck or shoulders. The closer the leg is to the floor, the more effort the abdominal muscles will have to make. However, if the lower back starts to arch off the floor or the abs begin to quiver, you are putting a strain on the back. Try again with the leg higher, but if you feel any discomfort stop immediately.

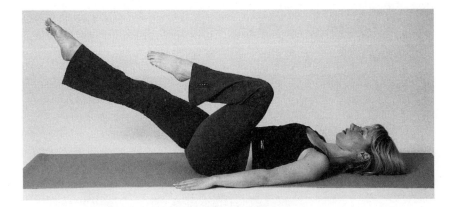

Take another long full breath and, as you breathe out, change the legs so the right leg is drawn in towards the chest and the left is stretched out. Always keep the whole back on the floor. Alternate 5–10 times on each side.

Alternate Arm and Leg Stretches

This exercise works on the whole central girdle of strength, with the added bonus of toning and stretching the arms and legs. The pillow is there to remind you to keep lifting the abdominal muscles away from the floor – when you get stronger, a gap should open up between you and the cushion – and you should keep it there throughout the exercise.

Lie face down with a cushion under the abdominal muscles. Stretch your arms above your head, with your shoulders relaxed and palms facing the floor. Place your feet a hip-width apart, the knees facing the floor. Breathe in and, as you breathe out, draw the navel to the spine and hold this position throughout.

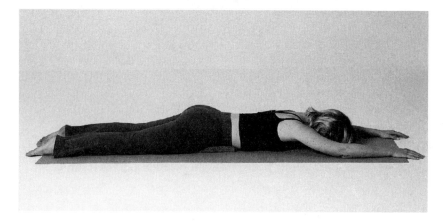

Breathe in and, as you breathe out, stretch out the right arm and the left leg as far as you can, keeping them low to the floor. When you have stretched as much as possible, breathe in and lower them to the floor.

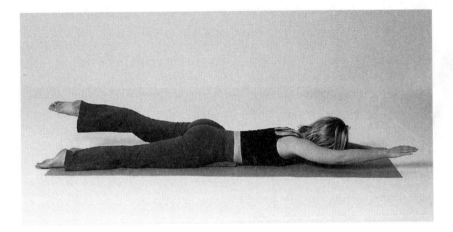

Breathe in and, as you breathe out, stretch the left arm and the right leg as far as you can. Check that there is no tension in the neck, shoulders or jaw and that the navel is still strong and drawn to the spine. Then repeat up to five times. Relax in the Child's Pose (see page 38) before going on to the next exercise.

The Hundred

This is a classic Pilates exercise in a simplified version – there is a harder one in Stage Three! Build up to this gradually. Don't expect to get to 100 taps the first time you do it and watch out for warning sides – bulging abdominals or backache – that you are doing too much.

Lie on your back with your knees raised, feet flat on the floor and your arms relaxed by your sides. Check there is no tension in your neck or shoulders and place a small pillow under your head if that makes you more comfortable. Breathe in and, as you breathe out, draw the navel to the spine and raise your legs so that your knees are bent and your calves are parallel to the floor. Gently point the toes.

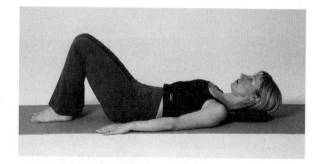

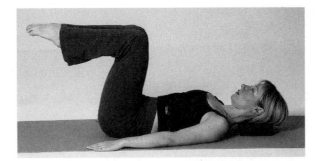

Keeping your legs in the same position throughout, breathe in and, as you breathe out, raise your head to look at your knees. With your arms parallel, tap your fingers five times on the floor on the next inhalation, then five more taps on the exhalation.

Breathe slowly and evenly and continue the taps in time with the breath aiming for 100 taps in all. If at any time you feel strain in your back, shoulders or neck, stop.

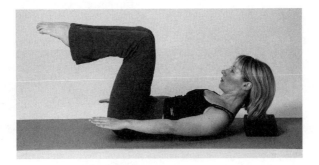

Draw your knees to your chest and hug them for a few moments, to iron out any tension in the back.

Stage Two Exercises 61

Leg Lifts 2

The added bonus of this and the next exercise is that they stretch and tone the legs as well as the abdominals. Make sure the effort is in the abdominal muscles and the legs and keep the upper body – particularly the shoulders and neck – relaxed.

Lie on your back with your legs stretched out parallel, with the knees facing the ceiling and toes pointed. Check that your shoulders are drawn down into the back and the arms are relaxed at your sides. Breathe in and, as you breathe out, draw the navel to the spine and keep your abdominal muscles engaged throughout the exercise.

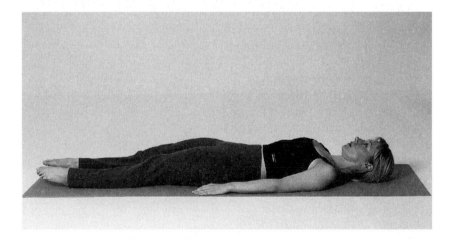

Pilates for a Flat Stomach

Take another in-breath and, keeping the navel held to the spine, raise the right leg to the ceiling and, if you are flexible enough, towards your body. Keep your leg straight and the toe pointed. If your back comes off the floor or starts to feel a strain, stop immediately.

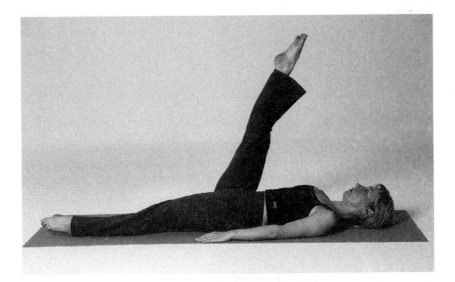

Lower the leg and repeat up to five times on each side. Hug your knees to your chest before you go on to the next exercise.

Oblique Leg Stretches

This exercise is a variation on single leg stretches that uses the oblique abdominals. Because there is a tendency to use the obliques least of all the abdominal muscles, this can be quite a tough one. If you find it hard, do fewer repetitions to start with.

Lie on your back with your feet flat on the floor and your knees raised. Breathe in and, as you breathe out, draw your knees to your chest and check that your back is flat on the floor and your neck and shoulders are relaxed. Place your hands loosely behind your head.

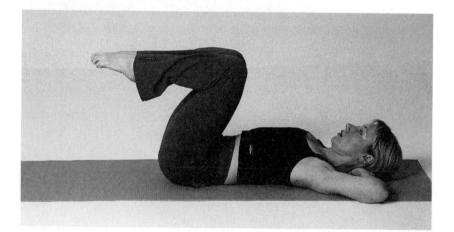

On the next out-breath, draw the navel to the spine and lift your head up so you are looking at your knees. Now stretch out the right leg in front of you with a pointed toe and turn the upper body so that your right elbow is reaching towards your left knee. The closer the outstretched leg is to the floor, the more effort the abdominal muscles will have to make – so take it higher if the lower back starts to arch off the floor or the abs begin to quiver. If you still feel any discomfort stop immediately.

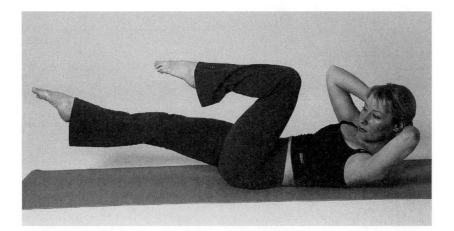

Breathing slowly and rhythmically, change the legs so the left leg stretches out and the left elbow reaches for the right knee. Check that the effort is coming from the abs and that you are not tensing the shoulders or using your hands to pull your upper body into place. Alternate 5–10 times on each side.

Stage Two Exercises **65**

Leg Circles

Try to trace the widest possible circle you can in this exercise, using your toe as a pointer.

Lie on the floor on your back as you did in the last exercise but position your arms at shoulder height, relaxed on the floor. Breathe in and, as you breathe out, draw the navel to the spine and keep it held throughout the rest of the exercise.

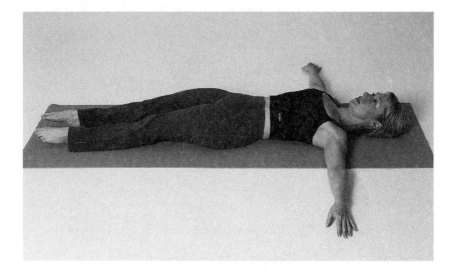

Keeping it as close as you can to the floor, take your right leg out to the side, as if you were tracing a circle with your toes. Inevitably, you will have to lift the leg off the floor at some point, but continue to keep it as low as you can while you continue with the circle.

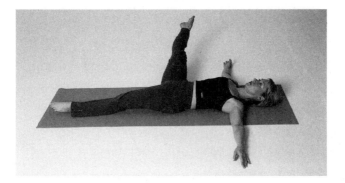

When the leg has come up as far as it can, take it across the body, still keeping the circle as wide as possible. Try to keep as much of your back as possible in contact with the floor. Complete the circle until the leg crosses back to the starting position. Repeat twice, alternating the legs.

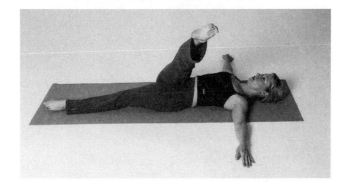

Contractions

The contraction is a movement from contemporary dance. It includes a pelvic tilt but works the whole abdominal area much more deeply as you draw it towards the spine. This has the effect of rounding the small of the back slightly, as well as engaging the lower buttock muscles. The rest of the body – notably the chest, shoulders and neck – should stay soft and open.

Sit up tall on your 'sitting bones' with your shoulders dropped and your neck and chest relaxed. Place the soles of your feet together and your hands either on your feet or on your ankles, whichever is most comfortable when you are sitting up straight and not leaning forwards.

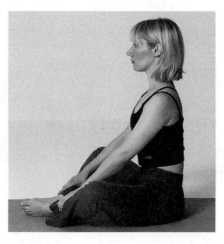

Breathe in and, as you breathe out, contract the abdominal muscles (all the way up to the top of the rectus abdominis, see page 3) so that you scoop out, gently round the back, tilting the pelvis and engaging the buttock and inner thigh muscles. Check that the shoulders and chest are still soft and open.

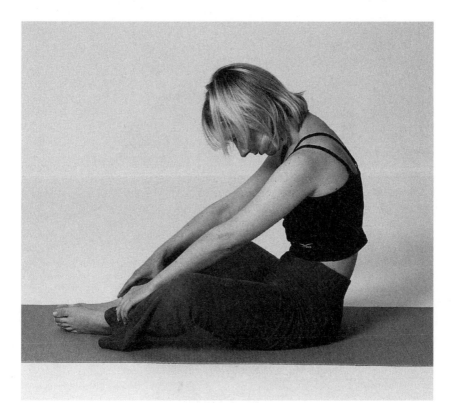

Hold this position as you take it forward in one piece, dropping the head down towards your feet. Don't worry if you don't come down very far – it's more important to keep the scooped-out shape.

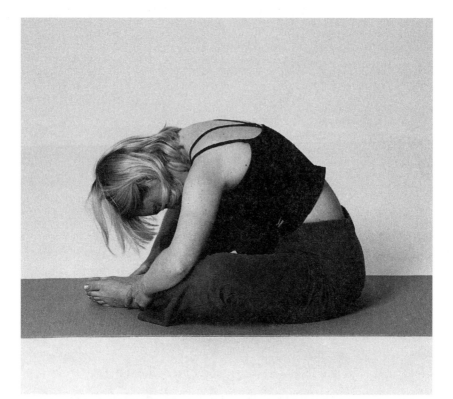

When you have reached as far as you can, breathe in and, keeping the hips exactly where they are, start to straighten out the back in a long, straight line. The line extends all the way through the neck to the top of the head, so you will be looking down towards your feet. Don't let the lower back round and check that the upper body has not tensed up. This movement is a long release of all the muscles and should feel like a stretch through the whole of your upper body.

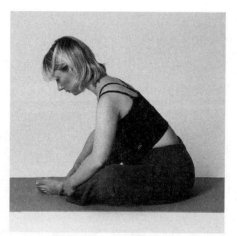

Holding the straight line of your spine, return to the upright starting position in one controlled movement, again without shifting the hips. You should feel lifted and taller than when you started. Check there is no tension in the neck or shoulders and repeat the exercise, slowly, four times.

Roll-ups

This exercise is excellent for building up abdominal strength, but if you find the effort goes into your back or neck, your abdominal muscles aren't yet strong enough. Concentrate on other exercises and leave this one until you're ready.

Lie on your back with your feet gently pointed, your pelvis 'in neutral' and your upper body relaxed. Breathe in, lift your arms and take them above your head and down on to the floor behind you so your fingertips and toes are now pointing away from each other in a long stretch.

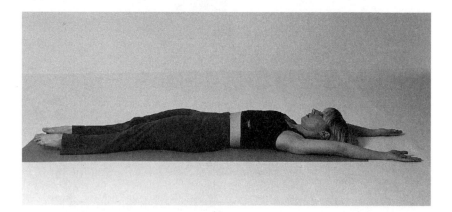

Pilates for a Flat Stomach

On the next in-breath, raise your arms to point straight up to the ceiling.

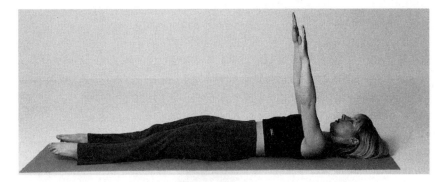

As you breathe out, draw the navel to the spine and engage the low buttock muscles. Starting with your head, the chin dropped to the chest, start to roll up slowly into a sitting position. The movement should be slow and controlled, with no tension in the shoulders, back or neck. (If there is, or if your abdominal muscles start to bulge out or quiver, they aren't strong enough – release back down to the floor.)

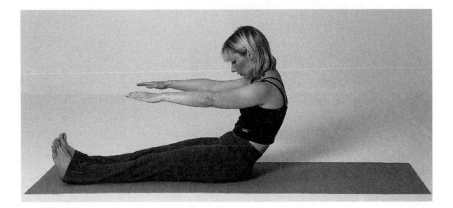

Keep your arms extended out in front of you as you roll forward, keeping your abdominal muscles working hard, the navel drawn towards the spine, so there is a rounded curve in the lower back. This will stop you collapsing over your legs as you reach forward.

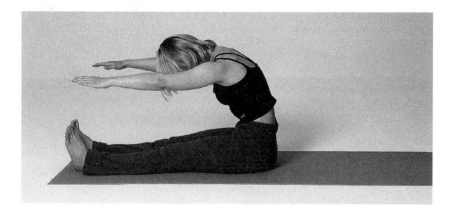

When you have reached your full extent, breathe in and, as you breathe out, roll back up to a sitting position. Breathing out, continue down to the floor in one long, slow, controlled movement. Repeat up to four times.

Finishing the Session

Finish off your exercise with the Cat (see page 34), the Pillow Squeeze (see page 40) and Relaxation Sequence (see page 42).

Stage Three Exercises

The final stage includes some very difficult exercises. If you have any back or neck problems, don't use these exercises at all – they will put an unnecessary strain on any weak spots you may have and you will achieve your aim more quickly and safely by continuing with Stages One and Two.

Build up gradually to the exercises, especially in the number of repetitions you do for each one. As always, stop if you feel any strain in the neck or back. It is a good idea after each set of two or three exercises to stop and relax the back, either by hugging the knees to the chest or by spending a few moments in the Child's Pose (see page 38).

Advanced Pelvic Tilts

This is a yet more strenuous pelvic tilt exercise. It is a good idea before you start to do some simple pelvic tilts as a way of mobilizing the back as a warm-up.

Lie on your back, knees raised with a cushion between them, feet flat on the floor. Check that there is no tension in the neck or shoulders and feel the spine long and flat against the floor.

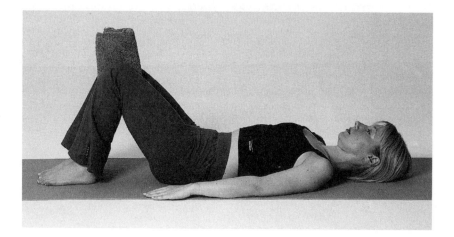

Breathe in and, as you breathe out, draw the navel to the spine, engaging the lower buttock muscles. Start to scoop out the abdomen and curl the spine up from the floor, vertebra by vertebra. Aim for a diagonal shape – don't push up too far or you will arch the back or tense the shoulders.

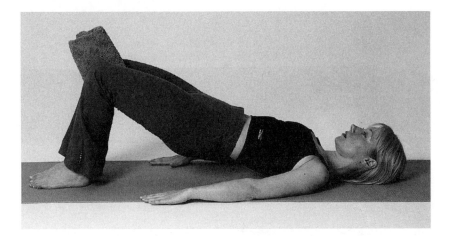

Holding your body in this diagonal shape – this requires some effort on the part of your abdominal muscles – and checking there is no tension in the neck or shoulders, breathe in and raise your arms. Lift them above your head and, if you can, place them on the floor behind your head.

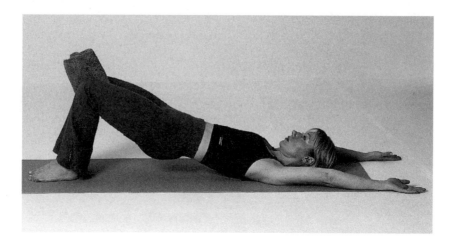

Pilates for a Flat Stomach

Keeping your arms behind you, breathe out and curl the spine back down to the floor vertebra by vertebra, making it as long and straight as you can. You will feel a strong stretch in the arms. Repeat up to 10 times.

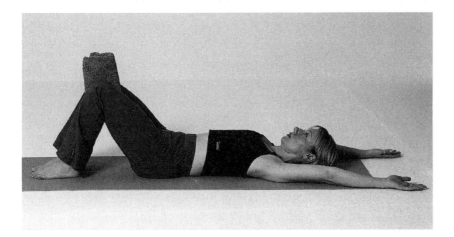

Curl-ups

As with the previous exercise, these curl-ups build on those you did in Stages One and Two, and are harder now that you have your feet up on a chair. Take them slowly and, if you feel any strain in the back or your abdominal muscles quiver or bulge out with the effort, you have come up too far, so take it lower until you feel stronger.

Lie on your back with your feet on a chair, your knees forming a right angle. Place a cushion or a rolled-up towel between your knees to remind you to keep your legs still and your hips level and check there is no tension in your neck or shoulders. Place your hands behind your neck lightly – don't use them to hoist yourself up during the exercise.

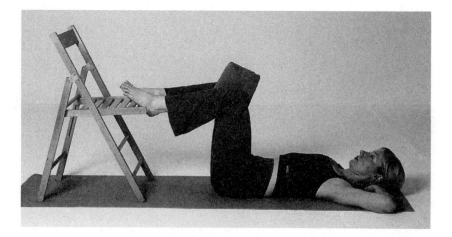

Breathe in and, as you breathe out, draw the navel to the spine, engage the lower buttock muscles and start to curl your head and shoulders off the floor. If you can only raise your head to start with, don't worry – just keep working at this level until you are stronger. The most important thing to check is that your abs are not bulging or quivering with the effort. If they are try the exercise lower. Another sign you have come too far off the floor is if the neck and shoulders start to tense up. The neck should be long, the shoulders down and you should be looking straight ahead, rather than down to your body.

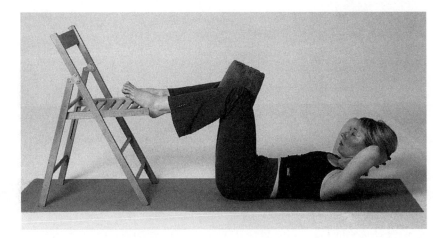

When you have come up as far as you can without straining, breathe in and roll down to the floor. Check for tension, especially in the upper body or the jaw. Rest if necessary and then repeat up to 10 times.

Oblique Curl-ups

As in the previous exercise, curl up only as far as you can without feeling the strain in your back or neck.

Lie on your back with your feet on a chair, as in the previous exercise. Check that your shoulders and neck are relaxed.

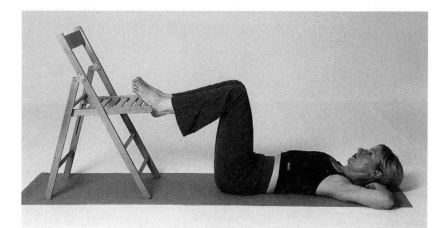

Breathe in and, as you breathe out, draw the navel to the spine, engage the lower buttock muscles and curl up, taking your right shoulder towards your left knee. As in the previous exercise, if the abdominal muscles start to bulge or quiver, if there is any strain in the back or tension in the neck or shoulders, you are coming up too far from the floor.

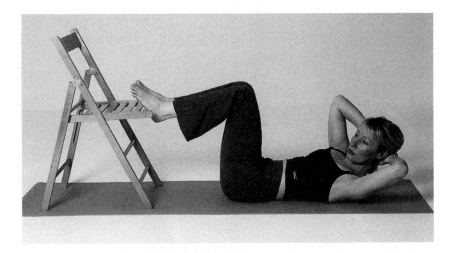

Breathe in and lower to the floor. Repeat on each side, working up to 10 repetitions.

Relax into the Child's Pose (see page 38) before you continue the session.

Legs Against the Wall

This exercise tones the legs, especially the inner thighs, as well as working the abdominal muscles.

With a cushion for your head, position yourself so that your bottom is touching the wall, with your legs leaning against it, toes pointing to the ceiling. If they will stretch effortlessly, straighten the legs and flex the feet, otherwise keep the toes pointed and the knees as bent as you need throughout. Do not arch the lower back.

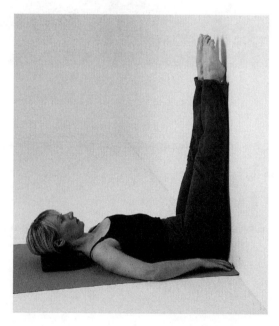

Breathe in and, as you breathe out, draw your navel to your spine and, pointing your toes, slowly move your legs outwards to the sides until you feel a stretch but not a strain. When they have reached as far as they will go, hold the stretch for a moment.

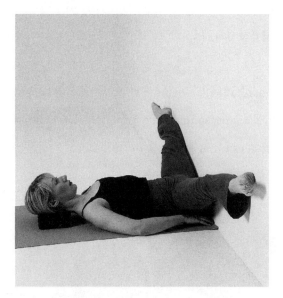

Breathe in and, as you breathe out, flex the feet and slowly draw the legs together. Keep the navel drawn towards the spine and don't let the lower back arch. It may look as if your legs are doing the work, but it is, in fact, your abdominal muscles that are holding their weight.

Repeat, flexing and pointing, up to 10 times.

Cat with a Leg Stretch

This is a variation on the Cat exercise that appeared in Stage One (see page 34). It is important to keep the hips level as well as the back flat throughout this exercise. If you find it a strain, especially on your back, do the original Cat instead.

Kneel down on all fours, elongating your spine and keeping your neck in line with it. You are aiming at a completely flat, table-top back! Make sure there is no tension in the neck or shoulders.

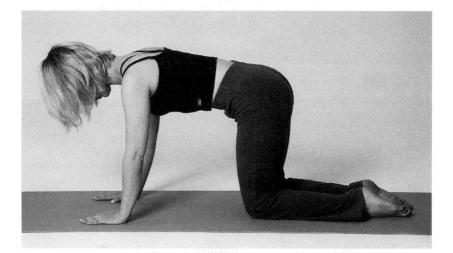

Breathe in and, as you breathe out, draw the navel to the spine and raise the left knee up towards the chest, dropping the head down to meet it.

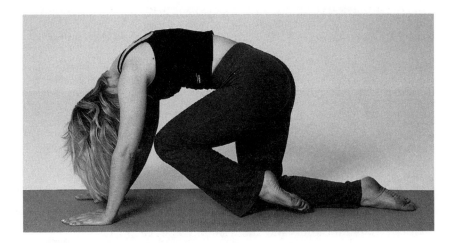

Breathe in and straighten the leg out behind you, raising the head back to the starting position. Repeat up to 10 times, alternating the legs each time.

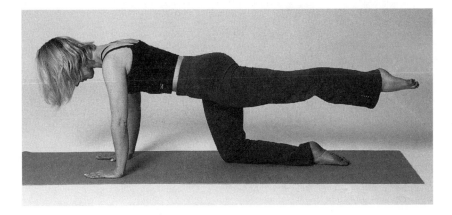

Side Stretches

This is a stronger movement than it looks as you are lifting the weight of both legs. It is important to lift them only as far as they will go without distorting the back or pelvis – watch out for rolling hips – or tensing up the shoulders and neck.

Lie on your side with your back against a wall, your legs stretched out in line with your back. Place your lower arm on the floor and rest your head on it, with your upper arm on the floor in front of you as support. Your face, shoulders, hips and knees should all be facing directly forwards. Check there is no tension in the neck or shoulders.

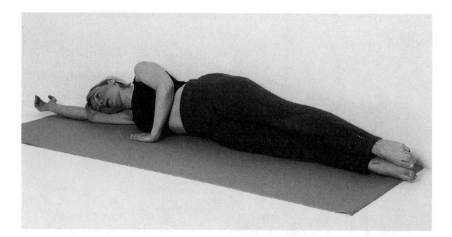

Breathe in and, as you breathe out, draw the navel to the spine, flex the feet and lift them two or three inches off the floor. The feeling is more one of stretching away with the heels than of lifting the legs high. Take care not to let the hips roll or the back come away from the wall.

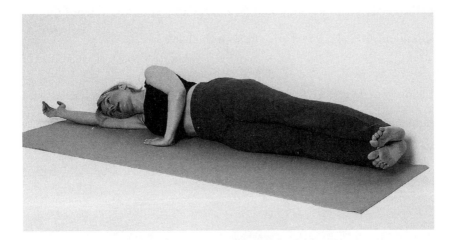

Breathe in to lower the legs. Check there is no tension in the shoulders or neck and repeat up to 10 times.

The Hundred

This is the hard version of the Hundred – and very strenuous it is, too, especially on the abdominal muscles! Work up to it slowly and go back to the version with the legs bent (see page 60) if you start to tense up the shoulders or neck, or feel any strain in the back.

Lie on your back and draw your knees up so that your thighs form a right angle to your chest, keeping them parallel and your feet pointed. Your arms are stretched with pointed fingers just a few inches from your sides.

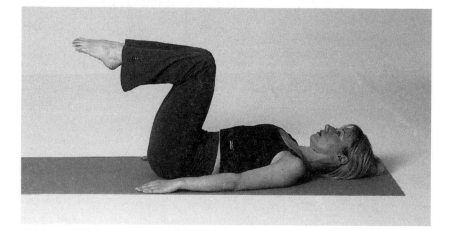

Pilates for a Flat Stomach

Breathe in and, as you breathe out, draw the navel to the spine and straighten your legs so that your toes point straight up to the ceiling. On the next out-breath, lift your head to look straight towards your thighs and lift your arms a few inches off the floor. Tap your hands on to the floor five times.

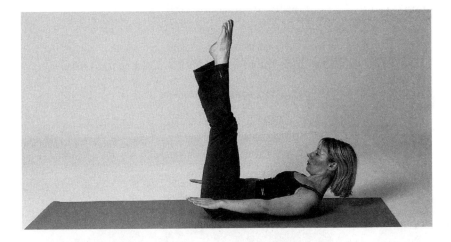

Breathe in, keeping the navel drawn to the spine, and make another five taps. Repeat, five times on each in-breath, five times on each out-breath, working up over time until you have reached 100 taps. If you feel tension at any time, bend the knees to a right angle or lower down to the ground and relax. However many taps you reach, always finish by lowering the head to the ground and hugging the knees to the chest for a few moments.

Double Leg Stretch

This is another classic Pilates exercise that takes a lot of strength, so work up to it gradually. Don't do this one if you have neck or back problems and, if you feel a strain in the neck or back at any time, lower the head back down to the floor and hug the knees in to the chest.

Lie on your back and bend the knees up to the chest so the knees are apart and the toes are together, the hands resting just below the knees.

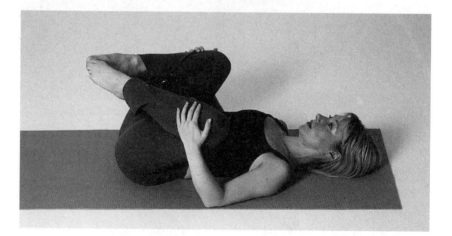

Breathe in and, as you breathe out, draw the navel to the spine and, without tensing the neck or shoulders, curl the head off the floor so you are looking towards your knees.

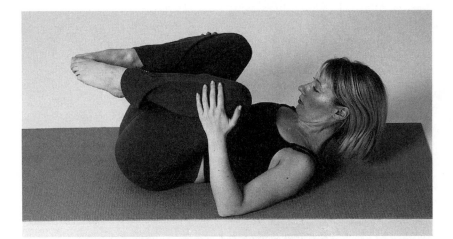

Breathe in and, as you breathe out, still firmly holding on to the abdominal muscles, straighten the legs and softly point the toes. Reach out with the arms so that they are parallel to the legs.

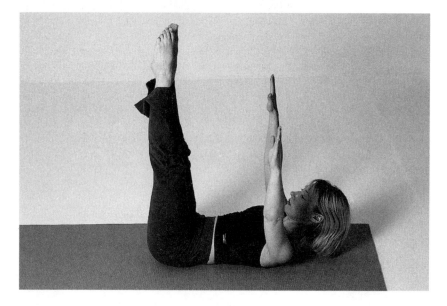

Keep the abdominal muscles engaged and the small of the back firmly on the floor as you breathe in. Turn out the legs from the hip sockets so that the knees face outwards – but make sure that you are turning the whole leg from the hips, not just the knees. Flex the feet if you can as this will extend the stretch in the legs, but if the stretch is too much, leave the toes pointed.

Pilates for a Flat Stomach

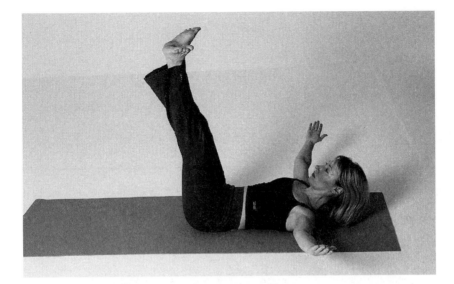

Breathe out and bring the arms up towards your face, behind your head and in a wide circle back to where they started. Again, check that your abdominal muscles are controlling the movement and your back is not arching or straining.

Breathe in, point the feet and lower the head to the floor. Bend the knees to bring the legs to their starting position. Relax for a moment. Over time, as you get stronger, repeat this exercise, working up to 10 times.

Crossed Pelvic Tilt

This is another variation on the pelvic tilt. Because you have one leg crossed over the other, you need to concentrate even more than usual on keeping the hips level and the back strong, without any arching.

Lie on your back, and cross your right knee over the left. Your left foot is flat on the floor. Check that there is no tension in the neck or shoulders and feel the spine long and stretched out against the floor.

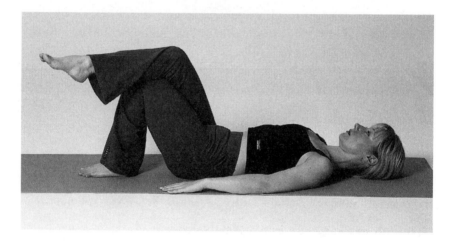

Breathe in and, as you breathe out, draw the navel to the spine, engaging the lower buttock muscles. Start to scoop out the abdomen and curl the spine up from the floor, vertebra by vertebra. Aim to get your middle back off the floor but not your shoulders. If this is too difficult, don't push up too far or you will arch the back or tense the shoulders.

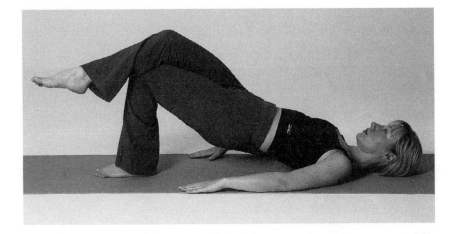

Breathe in and, as you breathe out, roll down very slowly until your back is down on the floor. Change the legs so that your left knee is over the right and repeat. Repeat up to five times on each side.

Forward Leg Lifts 1

This exercise not only works the abdominal muscles, it simultaneously tones the outer thighs and buttocks. It is vital, though, that you keep the abdominal muscles engaged as lifting the weight of your leg will otherwise place a strain on your back.

Lie on your right side with your back against a wall – this will help keep your spine in alignment and you will be able to tell immediately if you are arching in the lower back. Stretch out your right arm in line with your body and rest your head on it. If it is more comfortable, place a thin cushion between your arm and your head. Bend your right knee a little and place your left hand on the floor in front of you as a support.

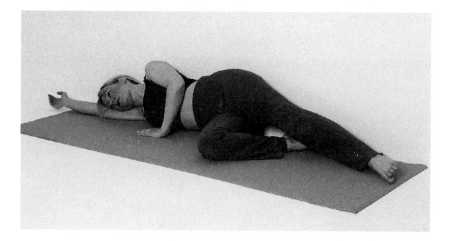

Breathe in and as you breathe out, feel your whole body lengthen. Don't let your waist slump down to the floor, but keep it lifted. If you prefer, you can place a small cushion under the waist to remind you.

On the next out-breath, stretch out your left leg with a strongly flexed heel and lift it a few inches from the right leg. The knee should be pointing straight ahead of you and this position starts at the hip rather than the knee or ankle. Turn your leg inwards in the hip socket for the right alignment.

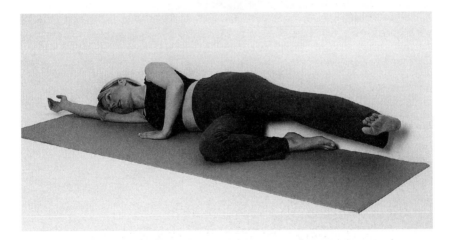

Breathe in and, as you breathe out, draw the navel to the spine and move your leg forwards so that your bring it – as far as you are able – to a 90-degree angle to the body, but still at the same height as it was before. Check that your hips are still parallel and there is no tension in your back or shoulders.

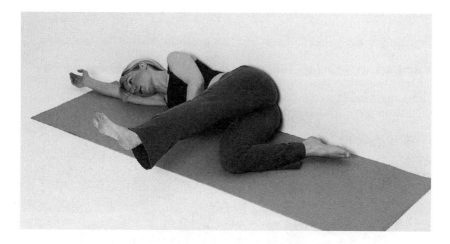

Breathe in and as you breathe out, return the leg to the starting position. Repeat this up to five times, then do the same thing on the other side, lifting the right leg.

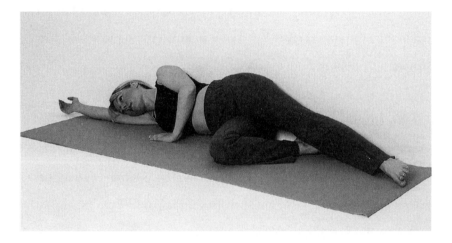

Forward Leg Lifts 2

This exercise is an extension of the last one. Again, watch out for tension in the back or neck and don't let the waist slump down towards the floor.

Lie on the floor on your side, with your back against a wall, just as you did in the previous exercise. Bend your right knee and place your left hand on the floor in front of you for support.

Breathe in and, as you breathe out, stretch out your left leg with a strongly flexed heel and lift it a few inches from the right leg. The knee should be pointing straight ahead of you and this position starts at the hip rather than the knee or ankle. Turn your leg inwards in the hip socket for the right alignment.

Breathe in and, as you breathe out, draw the navel to the spine and move your leg forwards so that you bring it – as far as you are able – to a 90-degree angle to the body, but still at the same height as it was before. Check that your hips are still parallel and there is no tension in your back or shoulders.

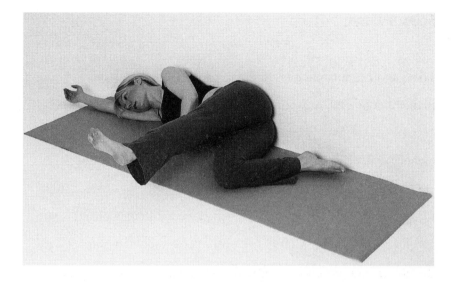

On the next out-breath, raise and lower your leg a few inches, keeping the leg straight and the heel flexed. Check that your back is not arching, your abdominals are still fully engaged and your neck and back are free of tension. Do eight slow lifts and lowers. Then repeat on the other side.

Scissor Legs

This is a very demanding exercise for the abdominal muscles. Remember that the higher the legs, though, the less demanding it becomes. If you find your back starts to arch or strain, take the legs higher.

Lie on your back on the floor, your legs extended straight ahead of you and your arms by your sides. Check your neck, shoulders and back are relaxed and your pelvis is in neutral.

Breathe in and, as you breathe out, draw your navel to your spine and bend your knees into your chest.

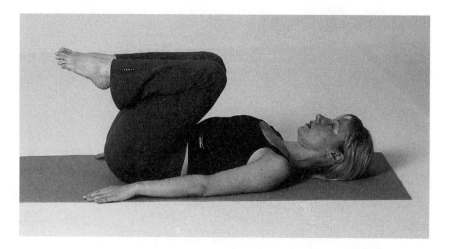

On the next out-breath, straighten the legs so that they point up towards the ceiling, toes softly pointed, and curl your head up from the floor, with your hands loosely clasped behind it. Don't use your hands or arms to hoist your head up from the floor – that will just cause you to tense up the neck.

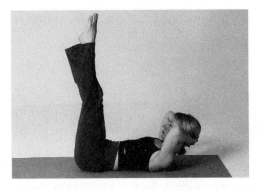

Breathe in and, as you breathe out, cross the legs at the ankles and then change to cross the other on top in a scissor action. Repeat up to 16 scissors. Hug the knees into the chest to finish.

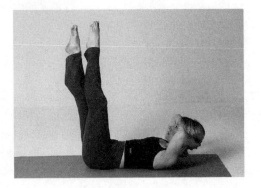

Contractions 2

This is another Contraction and it uses exactly the same movement as the one you did in Stage Two (see page 68). Now, though, you are sitting with your legs straight out in front of you and this requires more effort in both the abdominal muscles and those of the lower back. It stretches out tight hamstrings, too.

Sit with a tall, straight back, your legs straight out ahead of you, with the toes gently pointed. You should be sitting well up on your 'sitting bones', with the abdominal muscles gently held, your shoulders dropped and the chest soft and open. Check there is no tension anywhere in the upper body.

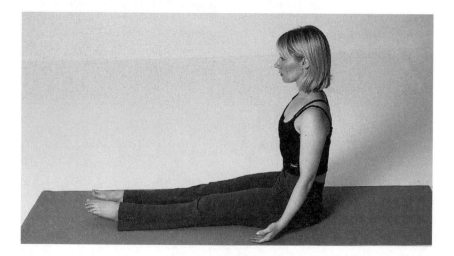

Pilates for a Flat Stomach

Breathe in and, as you breathe out, pull the navel strongly to the spine and tilt the pelvis upwards, at the same time as you push your arms away from you at shoulder height, with the heels of the hands pushing away too. Flex your feet and drop your head. The feeling here is as if someone has grabbed you by the waist and pulled you back at the same time as your hands and feet are being pulled in the opposite direction. So, there is a curve through the middle of your body, but you are not bending over towards your legs.

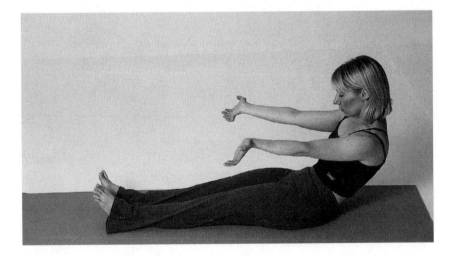

As you breathe in, release all the contracted muscles so that you extend your back and arms in a long, low (as far as you can) diagonal stretch, the feet and fingers gently pointed. The important thing to remember here is that your neck is part of the same long diagonal as the back – and both are still being supported by your abdominal muscles. Don't let the back curve or arch and don't let any tension into the shoulders. This part of the sequence is a release as well as a stretch.

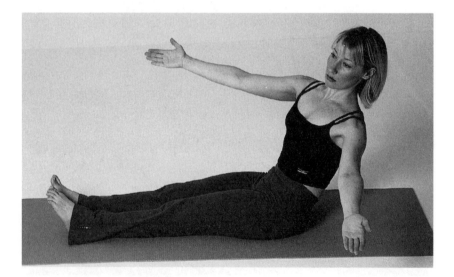

　　　　　　　　　　　　　Pilates for a Flat Stomach

Holding firmly on to the abdominal muscles, on the next out-breath, take your upper body back up to the starting position in one piece – without any curving or arching of the back which should be straight all the way through this part of the exercise. Check there is no tension in the back or shoulders and repeat the whole sequence four times.

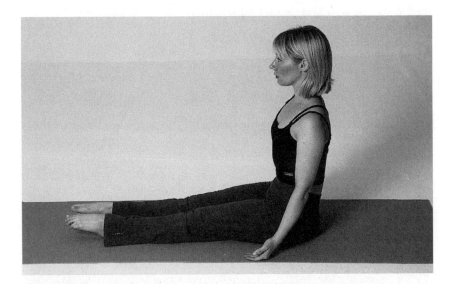

Pleadings

This is an exercise adapted from contemporary dance and again based on the contraction. It is supposedly named after the supplicating posture, though many dancers say that your abdominals have to work so hard their response is, 'Please, don't ask me to do any more of these!'

Lie on your back on the floor, with your arms by your sides. Check there is no tension anywhere in your body. Start with a pelvic tilt. As you breathe out, draw the navel to the spine, tilt the pelvis but don't let the upper body move. Breathe in and relax.

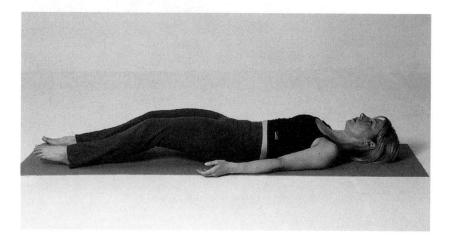

On the next out-breath, make the movement much stronger. Contract, drawing the navel back into the spine, engaging the buttock muscles in the pelvic tilt – this will cause the knees to bend slightly. Breathe in and relax into the floor. If you can do this without your abdominal muscles quivering or popping out and with no strain in the back, go on to the next step. If not, repeat the first two steps up to four times.

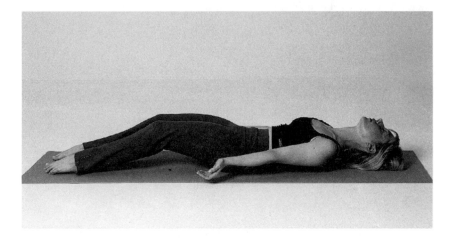

On the next out-breath, let the movement extend into the upper body, too. Contract the abdominal muscles, engage the buttock and thigh muscles in the pelvic tilt and lift your chest and shoulders very slightly off the floor. This can be a very small movement – it is a very strong one – but check that the top of your head is dropped back against the floor and your arms are extended out at your sides, palms up. Breathe in, roll back down and relax into the floor. Do the sequence up to four times.

The Rope

In this exercise, your abdominal muscles carry the whole weight of your upper body. The further you lean back, the harder it will be. You can do the exercise by leaning just slightly back from the vertical – it will still be quite hard! But don't lean further back to make it harder if you feel any strain in the back or if your abdominal muscles start to bulge out or shake.

Sit up with a long, straight back, remembering your neck is also part of your spine and should be in line with it, with no tension in the upper body. Your legs are long and straight ahead of you, the toes gently pointed. Engage the abdominal muscles to support your back – they should feel lifted rather than tensed.

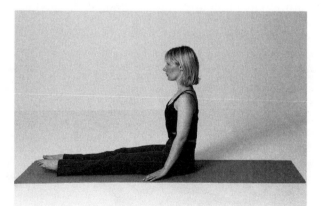

Breathe in and, as you breathe out, keeping the head in line with the rest of the spine, lean slightly back from the upright position, allowing your knees to bend slightly. Don't go any further than you can without straining either the back or distorting the abdominal muscles.

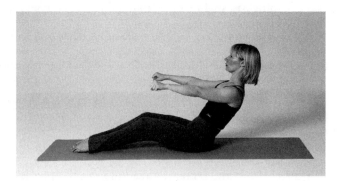

Hold this position and breathe normally throughout the rest of the exercise, making sure there is no tension in the shoulders or neck. Raise your arms so that they are extended straight ahead of you, in line with your shoulders. Make loose fists with your hands.

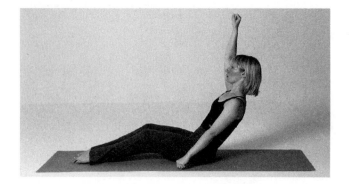

Now raise the right arm above your head, dropping the left down so that it is in line with your navel.

Take the lifted arm straight down in front of you as you raise the other, just as if you were pulling down a rope. Keep checking your neck and shoulders are not tensing up and that your abdominal muscles are not quivering or bulging. Keep the movement smooth and even, working up to eight 'pulls' on each arm.

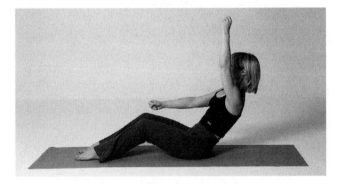

Put the soles of the feet together and drop the head down towards them, the hands resting on the ankles. Relax for a few moments.

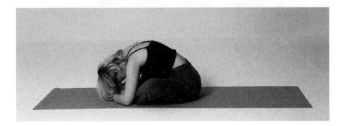

Arm Scissors

You are in the same position here as you were in the last exercise, with the abdominal muscles taking the weight of your upper body. Again, if it is too much of a strain, sit up closer to the vertical. This exercise has an added bonus as it tones your upper arms, too.

Sit up with a long, straight back, remembering your neck is also part of your spine and should be in line with it, with no tension in the upper body. Your legs are long and straight ahead of you, the toes gently pointed. Engage the abdominal muscles to support your back – they should feel lifted rather than tensed.

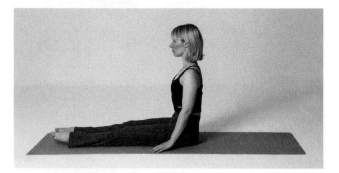

Breathe in and, as you breathe out, keeping the head in line with the rest of the spine, lean slightly back from the upright position, allowing your knees to bend slightly. Don't go any further than you can without straining either the back or distorting the abdominal muscles.

Hold this position and breathe normally throughout the rest of the exercise, making sure there is no tension in the shoulders or neck. Raise your arms so that they are extended straight ahead of you, in line with your navel. Make loose fists with your hands.

Move your arms slowly up towards the ceiling, crossing one fist over the other at the wrists as you go. Go only as far as you can without tensing the neck or shoulders. If you do feel a strain, drop your chin slightly towards your chest. If this doesn't help, sit more vertically or stop. Make four crosses.

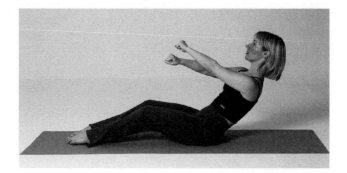

When you have reached your arms as high as you can without distorting your shoulders or neck, reverse the movement so that you take the arms down until your fists are level with your navel. Again, make four crosses. Repeat the whole sequence, aiming at four times in each direction, but always stopping if you feel any strain in your back.

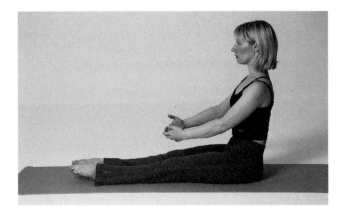

Place the soles of your feet together and drop your head down towards them, with your hands on your ankles. Relax for a few moments.

Can-can

It's not really a can-can, but you can see a faint resemblance in some ways. Unlike a can-can, though, this being a Pilates exercise, you move slowly and precisely, taking care to keep your abdominal muscles engaged and your lower back in contact with the floor.

Lie on your back, with your feet flat on the floor, your shoulders and neck relaxed and your arms by your sides. Check your lower back is in contact with the floor and there is no tension in your upper body.

Without moving your back, place your feet so that just the toes are in contact with the floor.

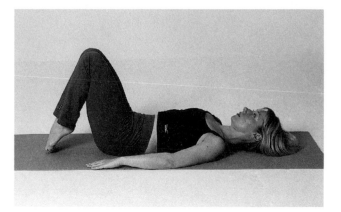

Breathe in and, as you breathe out, engage the abdominal muscles, tilt the pelvis slightly and raise the head just off the floor so you are looking towards your knees. Your arms, too, should come just a few inches off the floor, fingers pointing towards your feet. It is very important to lift your head only so far as it can come without distorting the back or bringing tension to the neck or shoulders. You can check this by turning your head from side to side and making sure it is relaxed.

Retaining the position above, straighten your right leg so that the toe points upwards. Replace, and straighten the left leg, checking with each change that your abdominal muscles are properly engaged and there is no tension in the back, shoulders or neck.

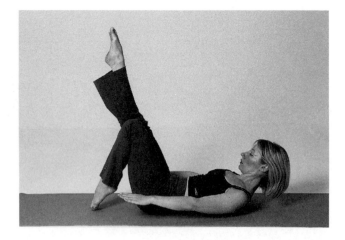

Pilates for a Flat Stomach

Repeat on alternate legs, up to 10 times on each side.

If you can do this with ease and without any tension or distortion in the body, you can try this with both legs – though, be warned, it takes a lot of abdominal control. Slowly lift both legs at once, and replace the toes on the floor. Work up to 10 repetitions.

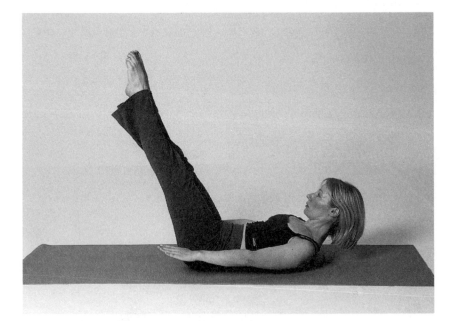

Seated Leg Lifts 1

This exercise and the next one use your legs as weights. All the effort in lifting them comes from the abdominal muscles. It is vital in this exercise that you keep your back straight – your abdominal muscles must be properly engaged to do this. If you feel any strain in your back, stop. You may find it easier at first to sit with your back against a wall, both as a support and also so that you can check there is no arching and you are keeping it straight.

Sit up very straight with a long back, remembering that your neck is part of that long, straight spine. Hold your arms in a rounded shape, with no tension in the shoulders and your hands just above your lap. Your legs are straight in front of you, toes softly pointed, knees facing the ceiling.

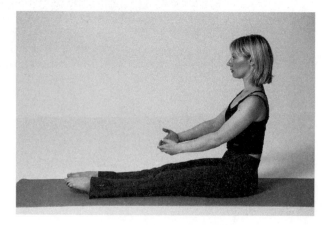

Pilates for a Flat Stomach

Breathe in and, as you breathe out, raise the right leg a few inches from the floor. Make sure all the effort of the lift is in the abdominal muscles, though you should feel the thigh muscles working, too.

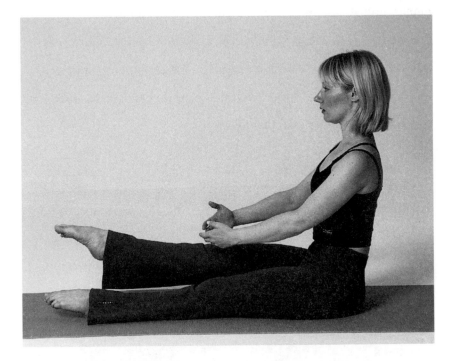

Breathe in as you lower the leg. Repeat up to eight lifts on the right leg, then repeat on the left.

Seated Leg Lifts 2

Remember that, just as in the last exercise, this one uses your legs as weights and all the effort in lifting them should come from the abdominal muscles. Again, it is vital to keep your back straight – so sit with your back against a wall, if that helps. It is also important to turn your legs out from the hip sockets, not the knees. Don't try to make your knees turn any further than the thighs can go.

Sit up very straight with a long back, remembering that your neck is part of that long, straight spine. Hold your arms in a rounded shape, with no tension in the shoulders and your hands just above your lap. Your legs are straight in front of you, toes softly pointed, knees facing the ceiling.

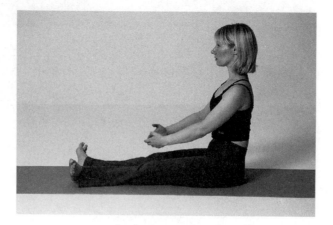

Pilates for a Flat Stomach

Breathe in and, as you breathe out, turn the legs in the hips sockets so that your knees face away from each other, and flex the feet back.

On the next out-breath, keeping the knee facing outwards, raise the right leg a few inches from the floor. Make sure all the effort of the lift is in the abdominal muscles, though you should feel the thigh muscles working, too.

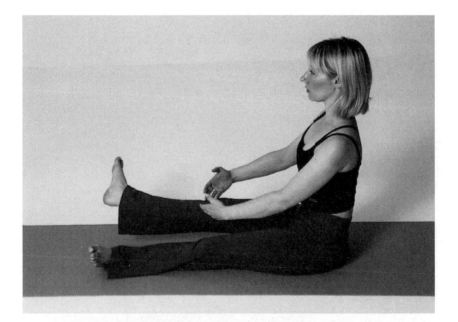

Breathe in as you lower the leg. Repeat up to eight lifts on the right leg, then repeat on the left.

Windmill Arms

As well as strengthening your abdominal muscles, this exercise also stretches out your hamstrings. It is important to keep your spine long throughout and to keep your chest open with no tension in the neck or shoulders.

Sit on the floor with a long, straight back, your neck and shoulders relaxed and your legs extended out in front of you with flexed feet as wide as you can without feeling a strain. Remember, when you start to move the stretch will be extended. Engage the abdominal muscles so that your back is supported.

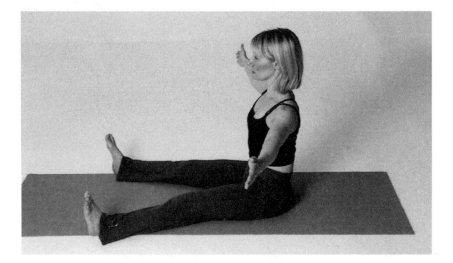

Breathe in and, keeping the back long and the neck and shoulders relaxed, lift up the arms until they are at shoulder height, the fingertips stretching away from you. Rather than lifting your shoulders to do this, try to keep them level. Instead, feel your shoulder blades drawing down into your back.

Breathe out and, keeping your hips and legs exactly where they are, twist your upper body to the left, controlling the movement with your abdominal muscles. Reach your right hand towards your left foot but keep the feeling of lift in the upper body – don't collapse over your legs to reach the foot.

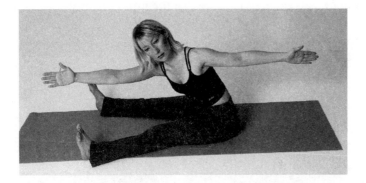

Breathe in to return to upright and then twist to the right, taking the left hand towards the right foot. Keep the movement smooth and lifted and the breathing even. Repeat five times on each side.

Foot Circles

Do this exercise as slowly as possible for maximum effect. It is important to keep the abdominal muscles and the pelvic floor muscles engaged throughout and to keep the hips absolutely level.

Lie on your back on the floor, your legs extended straight ahead of you and your arms by your sides. Check your neck, shoulders and back are relaxed and your pelvis is in neutral.

Place your hands on top of your hip bones and leave them there throughout the exercise to ensure that the hips remain still when you lift your leg.

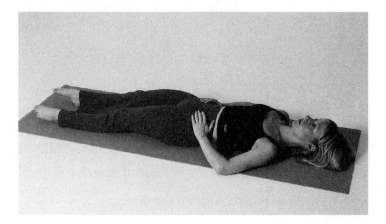

Breathe in and, as you breathe out, engage the abdominal muscles and the pelvic floor muscles and keep them held for the entire exercise. When you engage the abdominals, the lower back will come closer to the floor – it is important not to let it lift up as you lift the leg or the effort will be in the back rather than the abdominals.

Breathe in and, as you breathe out, lift the right foot a few inches off the ground, keeping the toes gently pointed. Make a small clockwise circle in the air, using your big toe as a pointer and moving as slowly as possible. Keep the knee facing the ceiling throughout and don't let your right hip move or your lower back come off the floor. Make 10 small circles clockwise, then 10 anti-clockwise.

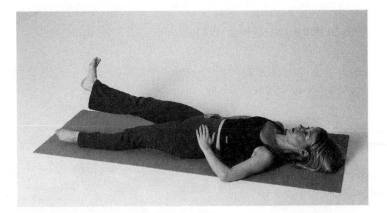

Repeat on the left leg for 10 circles in each direction. Relax on the floor for a few moments.

Shoulder Stand

The shoulder stand is a pose from yoga and it is a good way to draw your exercise session to a close. It improves the circulation, but you should not do it when you are menstruating. It is also believed to boost energy, concentration and longevity.

Lie flat on the floor with your legs together and your arms at your sides but with a slight gap between them and your body. Take some long, slow breaths and try to relax the spine down on to the floor and lengthen out the neck.

Breathe in and bend your knees towards your chest, so that your hips roll off the floor. Place your hands just below the hips to support them.

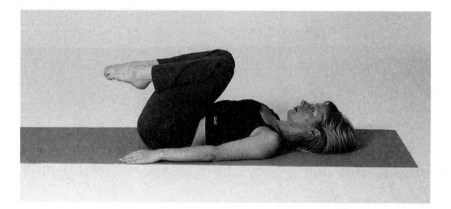

Continue to raise the legs in one smooth movement until your toes point to the ceiling. If this puts a strain on your back, bend the knees slightly.

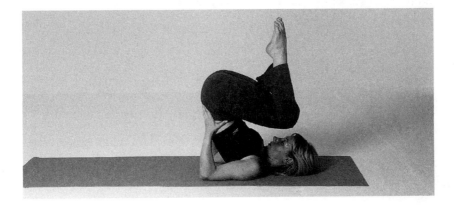

In this position, take some long, slow breaths, straightening your back and pressing your chin on to your chest – it is this action that stimulates the thyroid and parathyroid glands which may delay ageing.

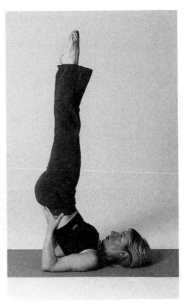

Follow the same sequence of movements on the way down and, when you are flat on the floor, breathe deeply and rest for a few moments.

The Plough

The plough is very similar to the shoulder stand but you may find it more comfortable to relax into the pose as it is less of a strain on the back. Alternating between the two poses is ideal.

Lie flat on the floor with your legs together and your arms at your sides, with a slight gap between them and your body. Take some long, slow breaths and try to relax the spine down on to the floor and lengthen out the neck.

Breathe in and bend your knees to your chest, so that your hips roll up off the floor. Place your hands below your hips to support them.

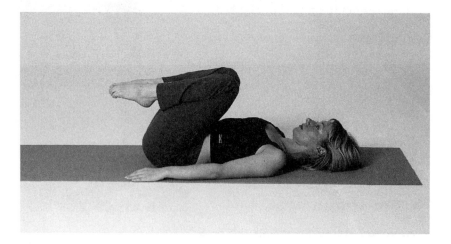

Breathe out and continue to roll off the floor so that you point your toes behind your head. Supporting the back with your hands, take your feet behind your head and, if you can, put them down on to the floor. If you find this position easy, straighten the legs and flex your feet so that the toes are curled under. This increases the stretch. Whichever position you are in, try to relax in to it and take at least five long, slow breaths.

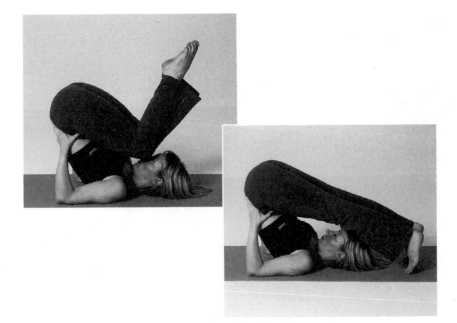

To come out of the pose, raise your legs, drop your knees down to your chest and roll the spine down slowly, finally stretching your legs out along the floor and relaxing for a few moments.

Finishing the Session

Finish off your exercise session with some relaxation (see page 42).

Pilates for a Flat Stomach

Day-to-Day Pilates

Pilates is not simply an exercise regime reserved for the studio or home workout. It is a system of movement that retrains the body out of its bad habits so that it can function at an optimum level the whole time. One of its most important effects is for posture. When you stand and move well all the time, you use and exercise the correct muscles automatically, both improving the way you look and reducing the risk of tension, strains and pains.

POSTURE

Posture is an old-fashioned word but it is of the utmost importance to all of us and by ensuring that your posture is good all the time – not just when you are exercising – every movement you make becomes a way of toning and strengthening the body.

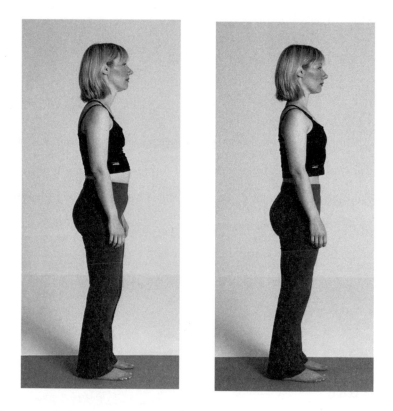

Many people have spines that end up in an exaggerated S shape and when this happens, pains and strains are not far behind. What you should be aiming at, instead, is the long but relaxed stance of a dancer. It is a good idea to check your posture not only before you start each exercise session but also in your everyday life. Stand in front of a mirror, preferably with another one set up to give you a side view, too. Here are the main points to look out for:

Head and Neck

The head should sit relaxed and balanced on the top of the spine with the neck long and in line with the spine. If you tip your chin up or jut it out, you will pull the neck out of alignment with the spine and this distortion will have serious consequences for your posture, creating tension in several muscle groups and, quite possibly, headaches. The chin should be tipped very slightly down to lengthen the back of the neck and you should feel as if the top of your head is attached to a piece of string pulling you up and lengthening you out.

Shoulders and Arms

The shoulders and upper back often hold a great deal of the body's tension, much of it due to incorrect posture. All arm movement should originate in the muscles of the middle back beneath the shoulder blades and the shoulders themselves should not lift up just because the arms do. Lift the shoulders up to your ears and just let them drop down into a relaxed position – this is where they should be all of the time. The arms should hang comfortably by your sides, without tension. Looking straight at the mirror, check that the shoulders are at an even height – sometimes one is tensed and held higher than the other, especially if you always carry a bag on the same side. Turn sideways to the mirror and check that the shoulders are neither pulled back (which distorts the neck) nor slouched forwards.

Back and Abdominals

Stand sideways on to the mirror to check your back. Let your spine lengthen out, the tailbone dropping towards the floor. Draw the navel gently towards the spine and gently pull up the pelvic floor muscles so that you do not overarch in the small of the back and your bottom does not stick out. Using these muscles protects the back from strain and is part of the Pilates 'girdle of strength'. For a flat stomach, this is the all-important area.

Buttocks

When your navel and back are in the correct placement, your pelvis will tilt very slightly upwards. If you gently squeeze the lowest muscles in the buttocks, this will help you keep the right alignment.

Legs and Feet

Your feet should be a hip-width apart, the toes facing forwards, not turned out. The legs should feel long and pulled up without over-extending the knee, pushing it too far back. Feel the weight evenly distributed between both feet.

WAITING GAMES

When you are waiting for the bus or standing in a queue, you can activate and strengthen your abdominal muscles without anyone even noticing. This is a good way, too, to remind yourself to check your posture and how you are using your muscles.

1   First, check you are standing correctly, feet facing forwards and a hip-width apart, shoulders and neck relaxed with a long, straight spine. Tilt your chin very slightly downwards to elongate the neck.

2   Now, check you are breathing deeply, not just shallowly into the upper chest. Take a few long, slow breaths.

3   Breathe in and, on the next out-breath, engage the abdominal muscles, gently pressing the navel towards the spine and pulling up the pelvic floor muscles.

4   Breathe in and relax – but don't let the abdominal muscles go completely, keep them lightly held.

5   Repeat up to 10 times, letting the upper body relax a little more on each breath.

IN THE GYM

Once you understand the Pilates principles and make them a part of all your movements, you can use them in other forms of exercise, as well. Apply Pilates principles when you are running or jogging, whether in the park or on a treadmill, to ensure your back is protected. Make sure your abdominal muscles are engaged, and that your neck and shoulders are relaxed – people often tense up this area when running. Most important of all – keep breathing! Emphasize the out-breath rather than the inhalation.

When you are exercising in the gym, incorporate Pilates principles into the way you use the machines. Remember to use the breath. Breathe in to prepare, then use the out-breath for the effort. This is particularly important if you are working with any form of weights or resistance machines as a way of protecting yourself from strain or injury.

You can apply the principles in just the same way in any dance or exercise class. Simply concentrate on keeping the abdominal muscles engaged at all times and let them take the effort of strenuous movements. Check on posture regularly, and particularly when any strain is involved – make sure the neck and shoulders stay relaxed and you can turn your head freely from side to side.

TELL THE WORLD THIS BOOK WAS

GOOD	BAD	SO-SO

Make
www.thorsonselement.com
your online sanctuary

Get online information, inspiration and guidance to help you on the path to physical and spiritual well-being. Drawing on the integrity and vision of our authors and titles, and with health advice, articles, astrology, tarot, a meditation zone, author interviews and events listings, www.thorsonselement.com is a great alternative to help create space and peace in our lives.

So if you've always wondered about practising yoga, following an allergy-free diet, using the tarot or getting a life coach, we can point you in the right direction.

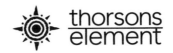

thorsons
element